Natural Alternatives to Dieting

*Why diets don't work – and
what you can do that does*

Dr Marilyn Glenville PhD

NATURAL HEALTH PUBLICATIONS

Natural Alternatives to Dieting
Dr Marilyn Glenville PhD

First published in the United Kingdom and Ireland in 2019 by Natural Health Publications
14 St John's Road, Tunbridge Wells, Kent TN4 9NP

Conceived, created and designed by Natural Health Publications 2019
Copyright © Natural Health Publications 2019
Text copyright © Marilyn Glenville PhD 2019
Artwork copyright © Natural Health Publications 2019

Production Manager: Chantell Glenville
British Library Cataloguing-in-Publication Data:
A CIP record for this book is available from the British Library

ISBN: 978-0-9935431-8-0

Disclaimer: The contents of this book are for information only and are intended to assist readers in identifying symptoms and conditions they may be experiencing. This book is not intended to be a substitute for taking proper medical advice and should not be relied upon in this way. Always consult a qualified doctor or health practitioner. The author and publisher cannot accept responsibility for illness arising out of the failure to seek medical advice from a doctor.

About the Author

Dr Marilyn Glenville PhD is the UK's leading nutritionist specialising in women's health. She obtained her doctorate from Cambridge University and is a fellow of the Royal Society of Medicine and a member of the Nutrition Society.

Dr Glenville is the former president of the Food and Health Forum at the Royal Society of Medicine and is patron of the Daisy Network, a premature menopause charity.

For more than 40 years, Dr Glenville has studied and practised nutrition, both in the UK and in the USA. She gives lectures and seminars throughout the world and appears regularly on radio and TV.

Dr Glenville has written 14 internationally best-selling books on women's healthcare which have sold over one million copies worldwide and have been translated into over 20 languages.

The Books Include:

Natural Solutions for Dementia and Alzheimer's
Natural Alternatives to Sugar
Fat Around The Middle - And How To Get Rid Of It
Natural Solutions To The Menopause
Osteoporosis - How To Prevent, Treat And Reverse It
Healthy Eating For The Menopause
Natural Solutions To PCOS
Natural Solutions To IBS
Getting Pregnant Faster
Overcoming PMS The Natural Way
The Natural Health Bible For Women
The Nutritional Health Handbook For Women.

Dr Glenville won the Best Nutrition Health Writer of the Year Award and has been awarded a place in the current edition of *Who's Who* of famous people.

Dr Glenville runs clinics in Harley Street in London, Tunbridge Wells in Kent and Dublin, Galway and Kilkenny in Ireland, and Dubai (see *Resources* at back of book).

For more information go to www.marilynglenville.com.

'Take care of your body. It's the only place you have to live.'
Jim Rohn

Contents

Acknowledgements

I would like to thank Hannah Ebelthite for helping to make sure that this book is easy to read. And to Donna Gambazza and Chantell Glenville for managing the logistics in the background.

I would also like to thank all the nutritionists who work with me in the UK (Birgitta Pain, Constandia Christofi, Anna Firth, Helen Ford, Miki Johnson, Sally Milne, Annabelle Patmore and Sharon Pitt), those in Ireland headed by Heather Leeson and Ciara Wright and also Sorcha Molloy in Galway and Alex Chaston in Dubai. And to Jessie Anderson, my clinic manager, and her team Annabel Bolton and Lucy Fordyce and to Abeera Zaidi my clinic manager in Dubai.

Last but not least, my love goes to my family: Kriss, my husband, and my three children Matt (and his wife Hannah and their children Katie and Jack), Len (and Mel) and Chantell.

Introduction

This is not another diet book. In fact, it's not a diet book at all. It's an *anti-*diet book. I am a nutritionist with over 35 years' clinical experience and know from working with hundreds of people that diets don't work. In order to achieve permanent weight and inch loss, you need to have a way of eating that becomes a way of life.

In your heart, you do know the truth of that and yet you cling desperately to the idea that all you need is a new diet, the *right* diet, and the pounds will miraculously fall off – and stay off.

It's time we all woke up.

• Exploding the diet myths •

Which of the following statements do you agree with?

1. If you eat less, you will lose weight.
2. Eating any form of fat is unhealthy and must be avoided.
3. Snacking between meals will make you put on weight.
4. Foods that are labelled 'low fat' will help you slim.
5. You must stick to a reduced-calorie diet to become thinner.
6. If you skip breakfast you'll lose weight because it reduces your daily calorie intake.
7. You must exercise for long periods to lose fat.
8. Low-fat spreads or margarines are better for you than butter.

As a nutritionist, I can tell you that none of the above statements are true – they're all common diet myths. Surprised? Many people are. But a belief in some or all of these myths explains why so many people struggle to lose weight – and to keep it off.

In this book, you'll learn the simple truths about weight loss – and will find out how to lose weight simply, safely and, above all, naturally.

It's been said before, over and over again, but let me say it once more, loud and clear: **diets don't work.**

It doesn't matter what kind of diet it is – whether it's high protein, high fibre, low carb, low fat, alkaline, paleo or a juice fast – they all end the same way. Yes, you might lose weight in the short-term, but draconian diets or faddy regimes simply aren't sustainable. The moment you quit the diet or regime, you will put on all the weight you lost and often more besides.

So, you might wonder, why not try pills and potions, or take the plunge and resort to surgery? Sorry but, once again, they won't work long-term. All you will succeed in doing is spending a lot of money and running the risk of wrecking your health.

If you're one of the millions of people who is fed up with dieting, you're in good company. In fact, you are a member of what is probably the largest club in the world. The largest club with the unhappiest membership. Do you really want to carry on like this, on a crazy rollercoaster? Don't you yearn to break out of the endless cycle of dieting?

If you're a dieter, you're probably an expert on the subject. You'll have read every article going about weight control and you'll have tried every diet under the sun. Maybe you've joined a slimming club or several and perhaps for a few heady weeks or months, you've even reached your target weight. But, once you stop dieting and return to your old eating habits, you find that the weight piles on again.

I can show you a totally different approach. An approach that works. I can teach you how to lose weight and to keep it off – forever.

And, no, I'm not going to suggest a brand new diet or trendy regime or faddy plan. I'm going to offer you a lifeline – a way to get off the diet treadmill. This book is your 'get out of jail free card', – your chance to stop letting food rule your life and ruin your life.

There's nothing complex or difficult about it. And, trust me, it *works*. Follow the guidelines in this book and you will easily, gently, *naturally* give your body the chance to get back to its ideal weight.

The key word here is 'naturally'. By their very nature, diets are unnatural – they force the body into unnatural ways of eating, into eating unnatural foods.

I want you to start being kind to your body. I want you to make friends with your body and to rediscover how to work *with* it, rather than work against it. *Natural Alternatives to Dieting* is just that – a *natural* alternative. And one that works.

Why you shouldn't diet

It's not just that diets don't work; diets actually end up causing you far more harm than good, not just to your physical health, but also to your emotional and mental health.

Anyone who has put themselves through weeks or months of dieting; of restriction, of deprivation; knows how devastating it is when the weight stops falling off and the numbers on the scales start to creep up again.

The effects of diet failure are devastating. Failed dieters often suffer depression, lack of confidence and damaged self-esteem.

Fuelled by the desire to succeed, it becomes all too easy to try one diet and then, when that fails, to launch into another, then another and yet another in the quest to lose weight. Before you realise what's happening, you've become what is known as a yo-yo dieter, with your weight bouncing up and down.

It's disappointing and demoralising, but yo-yo dieting is far more damaging than that. It is incredibly unhealthy because it distorts your attitude to food and steers you away from a normal eating pattern.

This yo-yo effect fosters feelings of anger and resentment as food becomes the enemy. You can come to hate and fear food and, in extreme cases, this can result in eating disorders such as anorexia and bulimia. In the past, it has tended to be young girls and women who were affected but nowadays men (and especially teenage boys) are also suffering from these terrible diseases.

Why we are pressurised into dieting

It's not surprising that we diet. First of all, there is an entire industry dedicated to making us feel the need to do it. The diet business in the UK alone is worth £2 billion[1].

Estimates in the US for spending on weight-loss products vary from $40 to $100 billion, which is more than the combined budget for education, health and welfare[2].

Slimming pills, replacement drinks, gimmicks such as fat-attraction pills, low-cal this, low-fat that – they're all big profit makers. Is it cynical to assume that the last thing the diet industry wants is for people to succeed in their diets and then stay slim? Not at all. Like all successful businesses, the slimming industry needs repeat customers. The media feeds and supports this industry with endless magazine articles about weight loss, image makeovers, make-up, cosmetic surgery and anti-ageing creams. The result is huge societal pressure on us to look good – and 'good' means 'thin'.

It's not just women nowadays, it's men, too. Every time we turn on the TV or watch a film, we see actors and actresses with perfect bodies and perfect faces. We're constantly shown images of how society views a perfect body. It's the same in magazines, on websites and across the ever-expanding world of social media. Fashion demands that models be a highly unusual shape (very tall but absolutely tiny in body shape), so that clothes hang in the way the designers want. Not only are we faced with pictures of people who are often unnaturally thin, the images are frequently manipulated to remove blemishes, wrinkles or excess curves. These aren't true representations – they're idealised versions of men and women.

Throughout this book, I am going to help you think about what's realistic, healthy and natural for your body. Not for anyone else's body and certainly not for the body the diet industry wants you to aspire to, but for *your* body.

An ever-increasing nation

Do you need more proof that diets don't work? Despite the huge diet industry and our collective efforts to lose weight, we are actually increasing in size. Over 60 per cent of adults in the UK are overweight and it is estimated that, by 2020, that figure will rise to a staggering 80 per cent. By 2030, half of UK adults may be clinically obese[3]. In fact, most of the developed world has a weight problem, which is spiralling out of control.

We can blame this partly on our sedentary lifestyle. In the past, most of us were active in everyday life but now huge numbers of us earn our living sitting at a desk and, when we come home, we slump in front of the TV or over a laptop. Certainly, this lack of exercise is a contributing factor, but the main reason for the rise in obesity is a huge shift in the type of food we eat. This has affected our health in general and our weight in particular.

If calories alone were the reason we put on weight, then we would all be thin. Did you know the Victorians ate up to 5,000 calories a day (the recommended level for a woman nowadays is 2,000 and 2,500 for men)? And yet they remained slim, so this challenges the traditional view that weight is always linked to calorie intake. So what's going on? The Victorian's were more physically active than us, but research also suggests their diet was very different from ours – refined, convenience and junk foods didn't exist[4].

Nowadays, of course, we have these types of food in abundance and each generation is eating more of it than the one before. Researchers have found that fat and thin people eat roughly the same number of calories, but fat people eat a different type of food from thin people – can you guess which type?

This book will explain which foods are best for your body. It will introduce you to a way of eating which is delicious and nourishing, while allowing your weight to reduce naturally over time and then remain stable. It will also help you to banish food cravings and say goodbye to food-related mood swings. It will advise you on shopping for food, preparing meals to eat at home with your family and will also encourage you to eat out in restaurants sometimes and have a normal social life. It's all about discovering a way of eating that you can maintain and enjoy. Natural eating, natural weight loss. A natural plan that will get you to your ideal weight and allow you to stay there... permanently.

Once you have the secret of easy, natural weight loss, you will no longer need all the specialist foods and shakes. You won't need to pay membership to slimming clubs. You won't need to keep buying one diet book after another. This book will reveal the secrets to successful, sustainable, natural weight loss. It promises to free you from the endless cycle of yo-yo dieting and serial weight loss and gain, forever.

This is not just another diet book

The information in this book is gimmick-free. It will teach you a completely new way of thinking about food – you will learn that your body needs to work in harmony with the foods you feed it. Any imbalance in the body's function can have far-reaching effects. But, equally, by giving your body exactly the foods it needs for optimum functioning, you will not just become slim and healthy – you'll feel wonderful, too. Your skin, hair and nails will gleam; your energy levels will soar; your sleep will become deep and restful and you will also notice huge shifts in your emotional and mental wellbeing. Your mind will be sharper and clearer, your stress levels will drop and your moods will naturally become more balanced. You will feel great in body, mind and emotions. Just as nature intended.

It's not all about food. We'll also look at fitness, because exercise needn't be scary or intimidating. You'll find out how exercise can not only help you lose weight, and keep it off, it can benefit your overall physical and mental health. And exercise can be woven into your everyday routine in ways that you might not have thought of before.

Some people may find that, despite following the food and exercise guidelines in this book, they still struggle to shift weight. But rest assured, this book discusses how to work out what's preventing natural weight loss – such as certain health conditions or medications – and gives you the tools to overcome those issues.

So, this is liberation time! Ditch the diets and let's look at how you can become the person you've always wanted to be – easily, healthily, naturally. Let's start to eat to live, rather than living to eat. It's a major life change and it's hugely exciting. Take the challenge and prepare to discover a brand new you. You'll be amazed at the difference.

Chapter 1

Why Diets Don't Work

If you've felt that dieting seems like a losing battle, you're absolutely right. First of all, let's take a look at what happens when you diet. It's important to understand this as you will quickly realise why dieting is such a bad idea for weight loss. Don't worry, it's not complicated.

Basically, every time you diet, your body thinks it's going to starve and so it squirrels away fat. As you reduce your food intake as part of a weight-loss diet, your body immediately panics and puts itself on 'famine alert'. You're giving it the impression that food is scarce and, therefore, it slows down your metabolism to get the most out of the small amount of food it is receiving. So if, for example, you crash diet for a week and then go back to your normal pattern of eating, you will be consuming your normal diet with a slower metabolism. Your body simply won't be burning up calories so effectively, which means that not only will you swiftly regain all the weight you lost, but that you will most probably put on extra weight as well.

When your body becomes scared of deprivation, it automatically clings onto fat. With most diets, you will lose only a small amount of fat before your body's fat protection mechanism swings into action. In this state of perceived famine, your body will hold on to fat at all costs and, instead, will choose to break down muscle tissue and lose water.

So, the answer is pretty simple. If you eat little and often, your body will relax, knowing that food is plentiful. It won't feel the need to store any excess in case there is a shortage and it can keep your metabolism at a good level. We'll look at this in greater detail further on in the book.

Not all calories are equal

In the past, there has been a lot of talk about calories, about how we need to cut calories in order to lose weight. Let's take a look at this. A calorie, in scientific terms, is simply a unit of heat – it's the energy-producing property of food. The perceived wisdom has been the idea of 'calories in/calories out'. In other words, if the calories you take into your body through food and drink are less than those you use up by bodily activity and exercise, then you will lose weight. Conversely, if you eat more calories than you expend, you will put on weight.

Now this is certainly part of the story, but it's not quite as simple as that. Nowadays, we know that the source of the calorie is also an important factor in this equation. We need to look at where our calories come from – whether it's from fat, protein or carbohydrate. Not all calories are equal.

Food can be converted into fat or energy. So, either you store what you eat, which probably means you will probably put on weight, or you can use it up by exercise and activity.

Whether food is burned or stored is determined by a number of chemical reactions which are activated by enzymes. Enzymes are protein molecules that act as biological catalysts – they speed up the rate of a reaction that takes place in or outside cells. Enzymes, in turn, are dependent upon vitamins and minerals.

Not all types of food, however, are easy to convert into energy. When the body can't do this, it stores the calories as fat. You'll hear the term metabolic rate or metabolism a lot around weight loss – it refers to the speed at which your body uses the energy from food. So if you're gaining fat, it's a sign that your body is not metabolising food properly.

To recap, when you go on a diet, your body cannot distinguish between a diet and a journey through the desert. It doesn't know whether the small portion of food you have just given it will be the last food it's going to get for a long while. So, its defence mechanisms step in and it holds on to any food it comes across.

A little bit *will* hurt

Imagine that you have been dieting for a couple of days and a friend brings you a cake. You decide to take a taste of the cake on the basis that 'a little bit won't hurt'. Once you begin to eat you find you can't stop and before you realise it you've eaten half the cake! Immediately, you find yourself consumed with a raft of negative emotions – guilt, anger, depression, self-blame, despair. But all your body was doing was fulfilling a simple and perfectly natural biological urge.

Put yourself in your body's shoes – it would be feeling deprived and nervous. It would be preparing itself for starvation mode and that slice of cake would have looked, not just appetising, but vital for its survival. The body would consider that the cake might be its last chance to stock up on vital calories. It triggered a cocktail of chemicals which are programmed to act on your behalf in terms of survival – so you craved more and more. Unfortunately, those same chemicals don't work on behalf of your waistline.

Trying to lose weight rapidly by crash dieting is going against all your body's programming. You simply can't tell your body that it's OK, that dieting will be good for it in the long term. Dieting requires you to be in a biologically *un*natural state in which energy intake is less than energy expenditure. Your mind and body quickly hear alarm bells and will resort to strong tactics to persuade you to eat normally.

Listen to your body

So, instead of crash dieting, try working in harmony and balance with your body and its natural hunger – you will be able to eat well, stay healthy and maintain your ideal body weight.

A study published by *the American Journal of Clinical Nutrition* showed that keeping our weight stable over long periods of time is linked with the best health[5].

It's fine to lose excess weight, but the problem is that (also termed 'weight cycling'); where weight is lost, then gained, then lost again and so on; more than doubles your risk of an early death and increases your risk of type 2 diabetes, high cholesterol, high blood pressure and increased risk of having a heart attack or stroke[6].

Why women have more fat cells than men

A man has 26 billion fat cells, or adipocytes, in his body while the female average is 35 billion. Fat comprises 27 per cent of an average woman's total body weight but only 15 per cent of a man's. This may seem unfair, but there are firm biological reasons for the discrepancy. Fat is essential for reproduction and, therefore, nature keeps fat stored on the female frame just in case a pregnancy begins. It is also necessary for ovulation – girls don't begin to menstruate until their bodies are composed of at least 17 per cent fat. Some women who take dieting or sports to the extreme over a long period of time find that they can't conceive or that their periods will stop if their body fat stores fall too low.

Because of this essential link between fertility and fat, the science of attraction means that men are inevitably hardwired to find curvaceous women more attractive because (even if it's subconscious) curves signify fertility and health[7].

Weight and the menopause

As the menopause kicks in, a woman's ovaries produce less and less oestrogen. Body fat becomes an alternative manufacturing plant for this vital hormone – oestrogen is vital as it helps the older woman combat the risk of osteoporosis. Your fat stores produce oestrogen throughout your life and during and post-menopause, body fat becomes even more vital to good health and it can be quite natural, and very healthy, to put on a few kilograms (around half a stone) over and above your pre-menopausal weight. This weight gain can start in the perimenopause, which can be anything up to a decade before your final period, as your oestrogen level starts to decline.

However, the balance is delicate: too much body fat post-menopause and you run the risk of having too much oestrogen in your body – a state known as oestrogen dominance. This has health risks such as breast cancer attached to it. But don't panic. As you work through this book, you will find how to get back in tune with your body, and discover the optimum balance of body fat to keep you at the healthiest weight you can be, whatever your age or life stage.

Being a healthy weight for your height (BMI - Body Mass Index - a ratio of height to weight) is very important in ensuring the post-menopausal woman has enough fat for the production of oestrogen. BMI is one of the ways to determine your ideal weight. Several studies have shown that BMI is a reliable indicator of osteoporosis risk. One demonstrated that compared with a BMI of 25, a BMI of 20 doubled the risk of hip fractures[8]. It seems that losing a significant amount of weight quickly may be particular relevant to loss of bone mass. So nature may have tipped the scales against women in their fight against fat but it has also worked in a protection factor – there's a good health reason why women find it much harder to lose weight than men.

Let's get realistic

When you diet it's not always easy to know when to stop. Dieting can easily become a way of life and it's possible to feel 'naked' or 'unprotected' when you aren't actively on a diet. Unfortunately, this mind-set can make you set unrealistic goals. Aiming to shed every last pound of what you consider excess fat makes the hurdle simply too high to jump, not just in terms of will power but, as we've just discussed, in health terms, too.

Remember those 'perfect' models? Don't even think about trying to emulate them. Very few women are naturally extremely skinny and, for most us, aiming for tiny dress sizes isn't just impossibly hard, it's a recipe for misery and lack of health. Of course, it's dangerous to be obese. If you're overweight to the point of possibly damaging your health then you must take serious steps to return to your natural, optimum weight. But how many of us are naturally tiny? For a start, not all of us have the bone structure and general body frame to be super-skinny – in fact the average dress size for women in the UK is 16 (the same size as the world's greatest sex symbol, Marilyn Monroe).

As nature has already determined your size, trying to be any smaller is probably a waste of time. After all, you accept that you can't magically grow taller – so why not be pragmatic about your width as well as your height?

Easier said than done, I expect. One interesting study looked at a random sample of 1,053 women, aged 30 to 74. It found that only 25 per cent were satisfied with their weight. A staggering 71 per cent of the women surveyed wanted to be thinner and yet 73 per cent of them were already a medically healthy weight. Many of those attempted dieting despite this[9]. How unnatural is that?

What doesn't work: popular weight loss methods under the microscope

Let's take a long, hard look at the many and various weight loss regimes that are out there. Most likely, you will have tried a fair few of them and might well be considering the others. My best advice? Don't. They all work against your body, against your natural weight-balancing mechanism.

All diets purport to help us lose weight but, let's be honest, if they worked why are there still so many unhappy, overweight women? Surely there must be one or two diets that actually work? The methods people have used to lose weight over the years fall roughly into three categories:

1. Popular diets in the media and used by celebrities
2. Surgery
3. Drugs

Let's look at the theory behind each method and analyse how successful (or rather, unsuccessful) they are – firstly in terms of weight loss and secondly in terms of actually being healthy and kind to your body.

1. Popular diets

You may recognise, or indeed have tried, some of the following diets. This list is by no means exhaustive – hardly a week goes by when I don't hear about some new fad. But it covers those you're most likely to encounter.

Very Low Calorie Diets (VLCDs) or meal replacement regimes

Very low calorie diets restrict calories to sometimes fewer than 500 a day – a quarter of what you actually need! This is usually achieved by using complete meal replacement. Some of these regimes provide the back-up support of a counsellor but in the majority of cases you're left to manage on your own. Replacement meals take the form of milkshakes, soups and bars. The replacement meals are designed to give the recommended daily allowance (RDA) of vitamins and minerals.

Verdict

These diets require a lot of willpower and by their nature are very boring. The weight loss can be dramatic but, by almost starving yourself, you can lose not just fat but muscle as well, which is medically unwise. To lose heart muscle, for example, is potentially fatal.

Many of these diets do nothing to change long-established bad eating patterns, nor do they offer help once the diet is over. Also, as the body is being starved, it will automatically lower its metabolic rate in order to protect itself. So, as the person returns to their normal eating pattern with a slower metabolism, more weight will probably be gained.

There are a number of meal substitute diets on the market, many of which can be purchased over-the-counter. Many VLCDs involve the replacement of one or two ordinary meals a day but some replace all meals and snacks so no 'ordinary' food is eaten while on the diet. VLCDs can work well for women who are busy and they do contain the RDA of vitamins and minerals but they should be used with caution. In my clinic I frequently see women with health-related problems as a result – in the main, they have presented with substantial hair loss once the diet is stopped and in some cases altered heart rhythms.

Food combining

This is an eating regime in which protein and starchy carbohydrates are eaten at separate meals based on the belief that these two foods need different enzymes to be digested effectively. The regime states that if they are eaten together, the food passes undigested into the intestines, resulting in fermentation, bloating and flatulence. After this, imperfectly digested food is not used as energy but, instead, becomes stored as fat.

The main rules of the regime are:

- Don't mix starchy foods with proteins
- Eat fruit on its own
- Don't take milk with either starch or protein
- Non-starchy vegetables can be eaten with either protein or starchy carbohydrates

Rules that are often added to the above include:

- High fat dairy foods should not be eaten more than once in five days
- One should cut down on wheat products
- Pulses (such as lentils) should be avoided because, in themselves, they combine protein and starch

Verdict

The theory behind this regime has not been proven scientifically[10] and yet there are people who feel the regime has helped with digestive problems (which in turn has helped them to lose weight). Critics often say that food combining works only because it restricts food intake and helps the person become aware of what they are eating. A theory based on the Glycaemic Index (see Chapter 2) suggests that we *do* need to eat protein and carbohydrates together.

High fat/no or very low carbohydrate ketogenic diets

This kind of diet has been around since the 1970s and has returned in a number of different guises since then, with some celebrities swearing by its ability to promote quick weight loss. One of the older versions of the ketogenic diet was the Atkins Diet. These days it's often called the keto diet or Banting.

It is based on eating high amount of fat and some protein such as meat and eggs but no, or very few, carbohydrates. Even fruit intake is strictly limited because of its carbohydrate status.

The theory is that sweet and starchy foods make blood-sugar levels rise sharply. When insulin is raised, more of your food is converted into fat, and you begin to put on weight. So it's thought that by cutting out anything that prevents a surge of insulin, you will lose weight.

Initial weight loss can be good, up to 6kg (1 stone) in the first week, but a large part of this can be water loss, not fat. When you are eating carbohydrates your body retains fluid in order to store the carbohydrates as energy. But you lose this stored water when you cut down on the carbs.

When your body is starved of carbohydrates, it has to get its energy store from somewhere else. First it takes it the energy from a stored form of glucose called glycogen, found mainly in your liver and muscles. About 4g (0.14oz) of water clings to every gram of glycogen so you can lose a lot of 'water' weight very quickly.

It is only when the glycogen stores are depleted that your body starts to burn fat for energy. This takes about three to four days and the fat-burning state is referred to as 'ketosis'. Ketones are substances produced in your liver if your body breaks down fat for energy, because intake of carbohydrates is too low. This is effectively what happens during starvation – your brain has the ability to use ketones so that it can survive even when there is no food available.

With a ketogenic diet you would be getting about 70-80 per cent of your calories from fat, only 10 per cent from carbohydrates and about 20 per cent from protein – although a lot of the high-fat animal foods such as cheese and meat are also high in protein.

Verdict

The research suggests that, in the short term, the weight loss on a ketogenic diet will be more dramatic than with other diets. But the same is not true long-term. When different diets are compared up to one year, they're pretty much equal with the people on low carb diets losing only an extra 1kg compared to a low fat diet[11].

Even when overweight people are put into a very strict controlled environment, in a hospital, and put on a ketogenic diet compared to the same amount of calories (but with high carbohydrates) they do not show an increase in fat loss[12]. And recent research has shown that cutting out carbohydrates could increase your risk of early death[13]. Having too many (more than 70 per cent) or too few carbohydrates (less than 40 per cent) in your diet causes a higher mortality rate. The researchers studied over 15,000 people and found a low-carbohydrate diet; with more animal protein and fat from lamb, beef, pork and chicken; was associated with higher mortality. But if the protein and fat were from plants such as vegetables, nuts, peanut butter and lentils this was associated with lower mortality.

The conclusion? Moderate carbohydrate intake (around 50 per cent of your diet) is the healthiest.

There are other problems with low carbohydrate ketogenic diets in that they have been linked to the development of non-alcoholic fatty liver disease and insulin resistance[14].

You can experience 'keto flu' as you dramatically reduce carbohydrates and symptoms can be fatigue, light-headedness and dizziness. This should go away over time, but ketones accumulate in the blood, causing side-effects such as bad breath (a fruity odour of acetone on the breath), poorer concentration, mood swings and bad memory. They can also create problems with mood changes, such as tension and irritability, resulting in cravings for carbohydrate-rich foods.

Another major problem is if the protein content of the diet is very high, excess nitrogen (a break-down product of protein) can build up in the body and damage the liver and kidneys. Protein also causes an acidic reaction in the body for which the calcium stored in your bones and teeth is a neutraliser. Eat too much protein and your calcium reserves can plummet, putting you at risk of reduced bone density and osteoporosis. In short? Steer clear of low-carb keto diets if you want to stay in good health.

Very low fat/no fat diets/hip and thigh diets

These concentrate on being so low fat they're sometimes no fat, which is a dangerous concept and one we will return to in Chapter 3. The dieter is asked not to eat fats;

including oils, nuts, seeds, oily fish, red meat, cheese (except cottage cheese), milk (except skimmed), egg yolk (egg white is acceptable), crisps and avocados. Poultry is allowed but all fat and skin must be removed.

Verdict

It's true that we generally eat too much fat. (The NHS recommends that we keep our saturated fat intake to no more 10 per cent of our total calories per day which is equivalent to about 20g.) Logic would suggest, then, that if we cut out all fat we are reducing our calories and will lose weight. But the question is, at what cost to our health? Certain fats, known as essential fatty acids (EFAs), are important for your health and it is unwise to go on a diet that eliminates them along with saturated fats. Your body cannot product these 'essential' fats (hence the name) so they have to be taken into the body via food or supplements. Totally fat-free diets can result in joint stiffness, skin problems and mood swings.

Essential fats are a vital component of every human cell and your body needs them to:

- Insulate your nerve cells
- Keep your skin and arteries supple
- Balance your hormones
- Keep you warm

EFAs can increase your metabolic rate, which in turn stimulates fat burning and increased weight loss. A good intake of EFAs is important, too, for those suffering with skin conditions such as eczema.

Few foods/mono diet

This diet comes and goes with different fads and trends. It usually concentrates on one or only a few foods. Popular versions have been the grapefruit only diet, cabbage soup or one where you are allowed six hard boiled eggs and six tomatoes a day. In other words, it's very restricted.

Verdict

As with meal replacement diets, these take the thinking out of what to eat and are invariably very low calorie. The diets will be low on nutrition and you could end up deficient in vital vitamins and minerals. Because they lack any variety they're likely to be difficult to stick to.

Intermittent or alternate day fasting/5:2 diet/16:8 diet

These diets have gained vastly in popularity over the past few years. The theory runs that by restricting calories on a number of days in the week (or hours in a day), you can not only lose weight but also reduce both blood glucose (sugar) and cholesterol.

There are many variations to this diet and nobody is clear which regime works the best. With 5:2 fasting you severely limit your intake on two days a week. However, it is not clear exactly how best to achieve this, whether the two days should be consecutive or broken up. Also, some say you should totally fast on the fast days (in other words drink only water) while others suggest 'fast' days should involve a limited intake (600 calories for men and 500 calories for women). It is also unclear whether these restricted calories should be taken all in one meal or spread out throughout the day.

Other regimes suggest alternate day fasting, where you fast every other day of the week.

During fasting periods, it is generally recommended that you just drink water but some alternatives suggest you can also load up on black coffee and tea or diet drinks to get you through the day (not a healthy suggestion at all).

On non-fasting days, no matter which regime you are following, you are supposed to follow a healthy eating programme but the temptation can be to eat anything and as much as you want.

Another variation on fasting is the 16:8 diet, where you fast for 16 hours and only eat within an eight-hour window. So in theory you could eat between 10am-6pm each day and then the fasting period also includes the time you are asleep.

Verdict

Intermittent fasting is strongly contraindicated for some people. If you are pregnant, breast feeding, have diabetes, are under 18 (and still growing) or have a history of an eating disorder then you shouldn't follow this regime. Also avoid it if you suffer from blood sugar swings (feeling weak, headachey, dizzy or light headed when you don't eat) I don't believe it is good for anyone suffering from chronic fatigue or stress (lack of food just presents further stress to body and mind), or those who are very active or in training for a fitness event.

This kind of diet is harder for women than men because women are much more susceptible to blood sugar fluctuations and these can be exacerbated depending on which part of the menstrual cycle they are in.

My major concern is that this type of fasting diet could tip some people into having an eating disorder. It doesn't re-establish a healthy relationship with food, which is really the ultimate goal for serial dieters.

I know there has been a lot of publicity and talk about intermittent fasting but at the moment there is very little evidence in humans to support the health benefits, including living longer. Many of the studies have been done on animals and those on humans have been conducted on small groups of people and only over a short period of time.

One study, which did take place over 12 months, took 100 obese people and gave them one of three eating plans. One plan restricted calories every day for the year. The second involved fasting on alternate days. The third plan was to just continue with their normal eating pattern. At the end of the study, both the diet groups had lost roughly the same amount of weight compared to those following their normal eating pattern, suggesting alternate-day fasting is not superior to daily calorie restriction. A high drop-out rate in the fasting group also suggests it's less sustainable in the long term[15].

Evidence is similarly sparse for 16:8 variation. A 2018, 12-week study compared 23 obese people eating only between the hours of 10am and 6pm to the group in the previous study who did alternate-day fasting.

Between the hours of 10am-6pm, the group could eat any type and amount of food they wanted and for the remaining 16 hours only water or, as the study says, 'calorie-free beverages'. Body weight and systolic blood pressure decreased for those on the 16:8 diet but other measures such as fasting glucose, fasting insulin and cholesterol (LDL and HDL) was not different from the control group.

The conclusion? There may not be anything magical about a 16:8 or even alternate-day fasting regime, other than a reduced period in which to eat and, therefore, a reduced calorie intake[16].

If this still appeals then I detail a much more sustainable approach later on in the book – the 12:12 (see Chapter 3). Already sounds more achievable doesn't it? It means eating within a 12 hour window and there is enough evidence to support its health benefits that I support its use as an optional part of my plan (note, I did *not* say diet).

Paleo/hunter-gatherer diet

This is another diet trend that has become popular over the last few years and, as with intermittent fasting, there are various interpretations that are followed.

It is based on the premise that we should be eating as in Paleolithic times, so it can also sometimes called the stone age, caveman or hunter-gatherer diet. And it involves only eating foods that could be hunted; such as grass fed meat, game and fish; and those that could be gathered from the wild; such as nuts, seeds, berries and most vegetables. It excludes grains, legumes (including peanuts), dairy foods, some vegetables; like potatoes, root veg, salt, refined vegetable oils and refined sugar; and processed foods, as they were not around in our ancestors' times.

Why no grains? The argument goes that they only entered our diets with the agricultural revolution (about 10,000 years ago). Because this is fairly recent in evolutionary terms, our bodies haven't yet adapted to digest them properly.

There are different versions of this diet, with some suggesting it is OK to have low fat dairy products and root vegetables that would not have been available during the Paleolithic era. Some say no fruit at all as it contains too much fructose.

But is all this *really* eating as the hunter gathers did? If you look at evidence from anthropologists, the answer is no.

The Paleo diet puts a heavy emphasis on meat but anthropologists have found that what most of the hunter gatherers lived on were plant foods and even the Hadza tribe, one of the last hunter gatherer tribes still living, get 70 per cent of their calories from plants[17].

Starch granules from plants and tubers have been found on fossil teeth and tools from as far back as 100,000 years, which has been suggested is long enough for us to have been able to adapt to them.

Our ancestors also ate a much more diverse diet than us (we know diversity is good for gut health). It is suggested now that 75 per cent of the food in the world is produced from only 12 plants and five animal species. And that of the 4 per cent of 300,000 edible plant species we only eat about 200 of them[18].

There are definite health concerns about meat (beef, pork and lamb), as it contains N-Glycolylneuraminic acid (Neu5Gc) which our immune system attacks, causing inflammation. Research has shown that long-term exposure resulted in a five-fold incidence of cancer and that consumption of red meat could be linked with other diseases such as 'atherosclerosis and type 2 diabetes which are exacerbated by inflammation'[19]. This happens whether the meat is cooked or raw. As Ajit Varki of the University of California and the lead author of the Neu5Gc study says 'red meat is great, if you want to live to 45'[20].

Verdict

Apart from the fact that I don't think this diet, if meat is going to be emphasised, is a good idea in terms of your general health, does it work for weight loss?

Large-scale trials to see whether the paleo diet works for weight loss do not exist. The only short-term study of three weeks was supposed to be done on 20 healthy volunteers (BMI less than 30) but only 14 people completed the study. And then the researchers only kept records and data on six people who showed an average weight loss of 2.3kg (5lbs)[21].

Plant-based/vegan/raw food diets

I realise your reason for following such diets may be ethical rather than for health or weight loss reasons, and they each differ. But I have grouped them together because they share many factors and they are becoming increasingly touted as weight-loss methods as well as lifestyle choices. With each of them, you need to give close consideration to your food choices to ensure an adequate nutrient intake if you're cutting out certain foods.

A plant-based diet may sound healthy but often people are living on white bread and lots of cakes and biscuits with added sugar. If you choose meat substitutes, they're often highly processed and full of sugar, fat, salt or artificial ingredients.

Vegans will need to ensure an adequate intake of vitamin B12 (found in animal foods), from fortified foods, yeast extracts or in a supplement. A vitamin B12 deficiency can give you symptoms such as fatigue, weakness and memory loss.

Iron can also be an issue as the most readily absorbed haem form of iron is only found in meat. Good non-haem sources of iron are beans, nuts, sprouted beans, cereals and green leafy vegetables – have them alongside vitamin C rich fruit or veg to increase the absorption of iron.

You could become deficient in EPA and DHA which are omega 3 essential fats found in fish oil (omega 3s are found in walnuts, chia and flaxseeds but in a less available form than your body needs to convert to EPA and DHA).

When it comes to raw-food diets, again I would argue they're not sustainable. We should eat according to the seasons and we are naturally drawn to soups and stews in the winter and salads and raw foods in the summer. And for certain foods the nutrient levels will increase with cooking, along with your ability to digest them.

Verdict

Research has shown that vegetarian diets are more effective than non-vegetarian diets for weight loss and a vegan diet was even more effective. But it is not known whether this holds for the long term[22]. One theory is vegetarian diets provide weight-loss benefits because they feature an abundance of whole grains, fruit and vegetables, which are rich in fibre and phytochemicals.

One study compared the effects of five different diets on overweight adults over six months – vegan, vegetarian, pesco-vegetarian, semi-vegetarian and omnivorous diets. All five diets were also low fat and low glycaemic index (GI). There were about 12 people in each group. The vegan group lost more weight (about 4 per cent more) than the other groups over the six months[23].

As well as the weight-loss benefits, it has been found that a vegetarian diet versus an omnivorous diet gives health benefits including protective effects from heart disease and cancer. With the vegan diet, the cancer benefit was greatest. There were also significantly reduced levels of BMI, total cholesterol, LDL cholesterol, and glucose levels in vegetarians and vegans versus omnivores[24].

It sounds too good to be true but, before you turn vegetarian or vegan in a quest for weight loss, remember as I said earlier that it's easy to have an unhealthy plant-based diet. Even if you avoid animal foods and eat more vegetables you will not gain the health benefits if you eat unhealthier meat-free options.

One study monitored more than 125,000 vegetarians over a four-year period for changes in body weight. There was a significant difference in weight gain in those who ate a high quality vegetarian diet with unrefined grains, nuts, fruit and vegetables compared to those vegetarians who chose sweets, chips and refined grains and gained the most weight[25].

In short? If you're following a plant-based diet you need to pay close attention to your nutrition and make healthy choices – it's by no means the easy option.

Juicing

Many diets or 'detoxes' require you to eat vegetable and/or fruit juices, and sometimes soups and smoothies, for a set period. The biggest problem here is the lack of fibre – when you put fruit or vegetables through a juicer it extracts the fibre. Fibre is important for digestion but it also helps you to feel fuller for longer. A smoothie is better in that it is just the food blended up without the loss of fibre. While this type of diet can feel healthy because you're consuming vast quantities of vitamin and mineral-packed fruit and veg, you're also having lots of fructose so it's not healthy from an insulin resistance viewpoint. It's also bad news for teeth. And you'll be lacking the protein, fibre and essential fats your body needs for good health.

Verdict

If you lose weight in the short term through juicing, it's likely to be water loss and because it's a very low calorie diet. But that also makes it unsustainable. Do you really want to drink all your meals? I would defy anyone to stick to a juicing regime for more than a few days – and I'd actively advise against it.

2. Surgery

More and more people are turning to surgery in hopes of a quick-fix for their weight gain. Between 2006-7 and 2011-12 the number of gastric bypass operations increased six-fold (from 858 to 5,407), according to figures from the NHS Health and Social Care

Information Centre. The number of gastric band operations has also increased from 715 to 1,316.

While there may be a case for surgery in extreme cases, it should not be undertaken lightly. It is highly unlikely to solve your eating problem long-term, and it's very far from natural. As with any surgical procedure, the benefits must always be weighed against the risks that accompany any use of anaesthetics – and are greater in cases of obesity.

Let's look at how far some people will go to try to lose weight. While some of the following procedures are, thankfully, going out of fashion, weight loss surgery in general is on the increase, particularly fuelled by the stories of celebrities who have lost weight via the operating table.

Endoscopic sleeve gastroplasty

This is a new technique, replacing a procedure you may have heard of called stomach stapling. It has a similar benefit in that it reduces the size of the stomach but it is a non-surgical, less invasive technique. The stomach is sutured (stitched) from the inside to reduce its capacity by up to 80 per cent. It is performed with an endoscope (a tube with a light and camera at the end) through the mouth.

Lap band (also known as gastric band)

During this surgical procedure a giant silicone band is placed inside the body, around the stomach. It works on the same principle as endoscopic sleeve gastroplasty in that it reduces the room for food in the stomach, but is reversible.

The band is adjustable after the procedure to the point where the band is not so loose that the dieter feels hungry but not so tight that food cannot move through the digestive system. You would think this might retrain the patient to eat less in the long term but the evidence suggests not. Research has shown only 11.2 per cent of people with gastric bands actually achieved satisfactory weight loss and 22 per cent regained their weight or even exceeded it. The researchers concluded that a gastric band 'is not an effective bariatric procedure in long term observation'[26].

Stomach balloon (also known as gastric balloon)

This is a keyhole technique whereby a doctor working with a small camera inserts a silicone balloon into the stomach via the mouth and then inflates it with water. The balloon stays in place for up to six months before being burst and removed via the mouth. As with the previous techniques described, this makes the volume of the stomach much smaller, so less food is required to feel full.

Stomach bypass (also known as gastric bypass)

This surgery makes the stomach smaller (like the lap band) but it also creates a 'short' around the digestive tract, shortening the length of the small intestines that the food passes through. It gives both a feeling of being fuller quickly like the lap band but also means that not all of the food will be completely digested. Because of the altered digestion, nutrient deficiencies can occur including vitamin B12, folate, zinc, calcium and vitamin D. As with all types of surgery there can be complications such as the risk of infection, internal bleeding and a blood clot in the legs (DVT). This type of surgery is thought to carry a higher risk of dying compared to the lap band[27].

Liposuction (also known as lipoplasty)

Rather than reducing stomach size to restrict food and prevent weight gain, this is about removing existing fat from the body (so it won't have any effect on eating). As the name suggests, the fat is literally sucked out from under the skin (either using a laser or standard canula). The patient is usually sedated, although some surgeons will consider general anaesthetic. Side effects may include infection and numbness in the area. There is a very small risk that an internal organ could be punctured, which could prove fatal. Some patients have complained of being left with baggy skin and if there is a lot of fat removed, it may be necessary to perform further, major surgery to remove this. Of course, you would need to drastically change your eating and lifestyle habits to avoid regaining all the fat removed.

Conclusion: can surgery keep weight off?

Although these techniques can certainly help transform bodies in the short-term, sadly none of the methods outlined does anything to retrain eating patterns to control future weight.

3. What about weight-loss drugs?

Many desperate dieters have been prescribed medication by a doctor or bought over-the-counter dieting aids. Drugs for weight loss work either by suppressing the appetite or reducing the absorption of calories. Let's look at the most popular choices and see how effective (or not) they may be.

Appetite suppressants

Amphetamines have been popular drugs for weight loss for many years - they work by reducing hunger and food intake. They also stimulate the stress response and can be addictive as they give a feeling of euphoria. Phentermine was one of the most common amphetamines used as an appetite suppressant – its highly unpleasant side effects could include restlessness, dry mouth, high blood pressure and hallucinations.

Another drug called fenfluramine (and later one called dexfenfluramine) was also on the market and it was reported that if someone took fenfluramine together with phentermine (the combination was called fen-phen) then the weight loss was substantial. Unfortunately, so were the risks of side effects. This combination of drugs was linked to primary pulmonary hypertension where a heart and lung transplant was needed. In this potentially fatal condition the blood pressure in the arteries feeding the lungs was abnormally high. In some cases, the blood could barely get through, putting the heart under massive strain. Fenfluramine and dexfenfluramine have been withdrawn from the market (and from the NHS) in the UK but phentermine is still available but on prescription at private slimming clinics.

A number of other drugs have also come on the market that help to suppress appetite and then have had to be withdrawn because the benefits of taking the medication do not outweigh the risks.

Calorie reduction drugs

One of the main drugs that works by reducing the absorption of calories is orlistat which is available both on prescription and over the counter in pharmacies in the UK. The one that is sold over the counter has the brand name Alli and is a lower strength than the one on prescription. This drug works by stopping fat being broken down and absorbed in the body by inhibiting an enzyme called lipase. Instead of the fat being digested, it is excreted. Average weight loss (alongside diet and exercise) is usually around 5-7lbs (2-3kg) more over a year compared to those not taking the drug, so it's not remarkable.

Longer term studies over four years show that weight loss combined with lifestyle changes on the orlistat is about 5.87kg compared to 3kg on the placebo[28]. Because excess fat goes straight through the body, dieters are asked to eat a low-fat diet otherwise they can get diarrhoea. Some pretty undesirable side effects can include anal leakage, flatulence and bowel pain. And many of the studies show a large dropout rate because of the side effects[29].

Taking the drug may also prevent absorption of certain important nutrients, especially the fat soluble vitamins such as vitamins A, D, E and K so it is suggested patients take a food supplement while on the drug.

'Natural' products

There are countless so-called natural products on the market that have been touted as weight-loss wonders. While these are generally not as worrisome as their chemical counterparts (although some are) I do have concerns with them.

Ephedra

This is a Chinese herb, also known as ephedrine and *ma huang*, which has been used in diet pills because it has a stimulant effect. It can cause an increase in metabolism but the stimulant effect also causes an increase in heart rate and increased blood pressure. These side effects have been associated with strokes and heart attacks. Other side effects can include irritability, anxiety, skin reactions, trembling and sweating.

Guarana

This is a plant which is found in Brazil. Like ephedra it is used for its stimulant effect, as its caffeine content is twice that found in coffee beans. Side effects can include anxiety, irritability, increased heart rate, sleep problems, dry mouth, heartburn and trembling.

Conjugated Linoleic Acid (CLA)

CLA is a type of linoleic acid found in red meats and dairy products and, when used in supplement form, it has been suggested that it can help with weight loss. The theory is that it decreases body fat and increases muscle but, whereas some studies have shown benefits on body composition, others have not.

Concerns have been raised that people with both type 1 and type 2 diabetes and people who are carrying excess fat around the middle and could be insulin resistant should not use CLA as it could aggravate insulin resistance.

Raspberry ketones

Raspberry ketones occur not only in raspberries but also cranberries and blackberries. But the level naturally occurring in the fruit is very low so generally it has to be made industrially in order to get a concentrated level of ketones that would have any effect on fat burning.

There is much publicity surrounding raspberry ketones and their ability to help you lose weight but looking at the evidence there has been no research on humans as to their effectiveness – so far studies have only been on mice[30].

Although the ketones themselves are not considered dangerous (but maybe ineffective) there can be side effects, such as jitteriness and anxiety. I would be especially careful if the supplement containing the raspberry ketones contains other stimulants like caffeine because the side effects can be stronger.

Why risk taking drugs?

Dieters will constantly look for a crutch to lean on, an outside influence to boost their flagging willpower. It's perfectly understandable but the more you diet and want gimmicks to help you lose weight, the more big business will try to give them to you. They make money while you fail. They provide the next fad and you pay for it.

All drugs carry some risk of side effects and so do some of these 'natural' products, so why take the risk?

Once again, just as with surgical 'solutions', you aren't really getting to grips with the behaviour patterns or food choices that most likely lie beneath your weight problem. Even if a drug or supplement seems to have an effect, that won't last when you stop taking it.

While I would strongly advise against it, if you decide you must have the support of a drug, then be sure to go to your doctor. Never buy drugs from the internet or from private slimming clinics, unless the latter thoroughly check your medical history.

My no-drug solution is simply learning to eat properly. And that is exactly what this book will help you do. Take control of your own body, your own diet, your own eating pattern and your own appetite. Truly, you don't need any gimmicky diets or drastic and dangerous surgery or pills. You can do it all naturally and safely.

But first, let's try and understand a bit more about how appetite and weight gain work.

What controls your appetite?

The hypothalamus is the area in the brain that masterminds the whole appetite process and hormones are involved, too. Ghrelin is the hunger hormone, produced in the stomach when it's empty and energy levels are low. It signals to the brain that we're hungry and our brain prompts us to seek out food. Leptin is the satiety hormone, produced by fat cells, that tells the brain we're full and so we get the message to stop eating.

Well, that's how it works in the simplest sense. But there are lots of emotional and environmental factors at play, too. Eating when we're bored, stressed or unhappy is not a response to hunger but a psychological cry for comfort. Our food choices are also determined by factors such as cost, availability, time available, cooking skills and our cultural background.

The pleasure we derive from certain foods can play a big role in how much we eat. Sensory properties such as taste, texture, appearance and smell will draw us to some foods and can make us eat more of them, especially if they're high in fat and sugar. When we eat for pleasure rather than nourishment it's easier to overeat. Then, if the foods don't satisfy us, we can end up eating even more. This is often called 'passive overconsumption' or 'mindless eating'.

Chocolate is one such culprit. It is not usually eaten for its nutritional benefits (although dark chocolate does contain some beneficial antioxidants). Its unique appeal has been linked to the aroma, taste and the texture (known as mouthfeel). And it's what can make us polish off the bar when we only intended to have a square or two!

Nature's delicate balance becomes distorted when some days we eat healthily but other days we stock up on junk. There may be times when we're too full to finish but somehow find space for dessert; then other times when you have overpowering cravings for certain foods.

Emotional attachment to food is tricky because we all need to eat to live. Unlike smokers who can just quit, it's not possible to go cold turkey on eating.

The health risks of being overweight or obese

We all know that being overweight is not good for your health. Carrying excess weight around can cause joint pain, arthritis and back trouble – because your body is having to deal with too much bulk.

But more severe health problems can be caused, depending on where you carry that excess weight. We now know that having fat around the middle increases your risk of a number of serious illnesses. (For very detailed information on this, read my book totally dedicated to this topic – *Fat Around The Middle*.)

If the ratio of your waist-to-hip measurement is more than 0.8 (for women and 0.95 for men), you may have a greater risk of heart disease, type 2 diabetes, high blood pressure, cancer (especially breast cancer) and Alzheimer's disease and you need to take preventative measures. To calculate your waist-to-hip ratio:

1. Measure your waist, finding where it is the narrowest.
2. Measure your hips at their widest point.
3. Divide your waist measurement by your hip measurement to calculate your ratio.

For example:

79cm (31in) waist divided by 94cm (37in) hip = 0.84

Being overweight or obese is linked to 12 different cancers according to the World Cancer Research Fund, including bowel, gallbladder, kidney, liver, mouth, oesophagus, ovary, pancreas, prostate, stomach, womb and breast.

If that's you, don't worry. The advice I'm going to give you in this book will help you bring your waist-to-hip ratio down, alongside your overall weight.

Fat loss not weight loss

When you say you want to lose weight what you're actually saying is that you want to lose fat. Looking at ourselves in simple terms, we are made up of fat and lean mass (including muscle). Researchers have found that when women diet, almost 25 per cent of that weight loss can comprise water, bone and muscle. People on rapid weight loss diets tend to look haggard because they are losing muscle tissue and not much fat. Crash diets with large amounts of weight loss may sound appealing but you simply can't lose more than 900g (2lbs) of fat a week healthily. Real, permanent, natural, safe and effective fat loss has to be gradual and yes, it does take time. But it works and the fat stays off.

The good news

My aim in this chapter was not to dishearten you, but to show you why all the quick fixes and wonder diets and regimes, all the pills and potions, all the surgeries and, yes, so-called natural super supplements, won't help you with long-term weight loss.

But now, it's time for the good news. There *is* a way you can lose weight, as much weight as you need to. Even better, I am not going to suggest that you starve yourself. Far from it. In fact, one of the most surprising things you'll learn in this book is that you may well not be eating *enough*. The eating plan I suggest lets you eat more, get healthy and still lose weight – lots of weight. You may be surprised to find that some foods can actually help you lose weight (and no, I'm not talking about wonder-pills but normal foods).

Ready to lose weight naturally and forever? Let's get started.

• Chapter 2 •

Mood, Food and Cravings

There's hardly a dieter in the world who hasn't experienced overwhelming cravings. It's always the same. You stick quite happily to your diet for days, sometimes for weeks, then suddenly all the good work is blown in one 10-minute eating frenzy. It's as if you have two voices inside your head. One says: 'You know you don't really need that bar of chocolate', while the other whispers, 'Oh, go on, a little bit won't make any difference'.

Of course, if you listen to the second voice it will never stop at, 'a little bit'. Before you know it, you've eaten the whole bar and maybe even a second one too. Your heart sinks as you step on the scales and then despair turns to anger. Your mind turns truculent and it reasons that since you've already ruined the day's dieting, you may as well give up and have chips for supper and finish off with syrup pudding. Sound familiar?

We know it's crazy. We know it's self-defeating and that, once we've given in to our craving, we'll feel guilty and depressed, so why on earth do we do it? Is it just greed that gets the better of us? Or is it something much deeper?

Greed or need?

Occasionally, cravings can be put down to greed but, to my thinking, that's too simplistic. Cravings are far more likely to stem from a biochemical urge that is almost impossible to control by mind power alone. Your body is demanding a particular type of food, usually sugar, because it has a need for it. And when your body has a need it will let you know in no uncertain terms.

Many diet gurus will tell you that the only way to banish cravings is to keep all tempting foods out of sight and out of reach. They will advise you to clear your cupboards, empty your fridge, put a padlock on the biscuit tin. When a craving strikes, they suggest you suffer through, using every last inch of willpower. But, as anyone who has ever experienced cravings knows, that is sheer torture. It is also totally non-productive. Not only will it make you feel angry and guilty, it will also foster feelings of self-denial. The dieter often ends up feeling useless, worthless and totally deserving of being fat and ugly.

Banishing tempting foods isn't the answer. It is much better to change your biochemistry so that your body simply won't have such uncontrollable needs.

Sounds difficult? Actually it is incredibly simple; so simple that you will wonder why nobody explained it to you before. Cravings are linked with mood swings, caused by biochemical changes in your body. Adjust your biochemistry and you will find yourself in control of those cravings. This chapter contains the key to controlling those Jekyll and Hyde mood swings – yes, even premenstrual ones. Without doubt it will help you on your way to successful weight loss – without cravings.

Get to know your blood sugar levels

Almost everyone who struggles with weight has an underlying blood sugar imbalance. Blood sugar – literally, the amount of sugar circulating in your bloodstream – can be the most important factor in losing and maintaining a healthy weight.

Fluctuations in blood sugar can cause:

- cravings
- water retention
- excess thirst
- mood swings

Does your mood swing from euphoric to depressed, almost from one moment to the next? Do you veer from angry to couldn't care less? From irritable and anxious to bored and tired? Blame your blood sugar. And know that positive highs can be just as dangerous as negative lows. Swinging rapidly from one extreme of mood to the other is a disaster for your weight-loss plans. You need to take control of these highs and lows because wild blood sugar swings will bring on food cravings and food cravings will, without a shadow of a doubt, undermine all your efforts to change your eating patterns.

How do you know if your blood sugar is fluctuating?

Answer the following questions:

1. Do you need more than eight hours sleep a night?
2. Do you find it hard to wake up in the morning?
3. Do you drink coffee, tea or soft drinks throughout the day?
4. Do you feel drowsy during the day?
5. Do you get dizzy and irritable if you don't eat?
6. Do you sweat or get very thirsty?
7. Do you lose concentration or feel forgetful?

8. Do you crave sweet foods or sweet drinks?
9. Do you have less energy than you used to?
10. Do you get angry or aggressive inappropriately?
11. Do you wake at 3am or 4am?
12. Do you often wake up with a headache?
13. Do you need to eat in the middle of the night to get back to sleep?

If you have answered 'yes' to five or more of the questions above, then it is very likely your blood sugar is fluctuating quite markedly and making you prone to cravings, mood swings and creating difficulties with weight loss.

This chapter is designed to make you more aware of what is happening in your body – at a biochemical level. You may already have made some connections – for example, that you are only overcome by cravings for sweet things at pre-menstrual times. This is your chance to look more deeply at the issue and to learn why your body does what it does. The good news is that it's not about willpower – it's not your mind's fault that you can't give up certain foods. It's simply that nobody has told you how to give your body what it needs – balanced blood sugar.

Let's look more closely at how blood sugar levels are controlled.

Nutrition and blood sugar

Nutrition is the key to stabilising the levels of blood sugar in your bloodstream. After a meal, glucose from the breakdown of food (digestion) is absorbed through the wall of your intestine into your bloodstream. At this point, there is, quite naturally, a high level of glucose in your blood. Your body takes what it immediately needs for energy and also produces insulin from the pancreas in an attempt to lower the level of excess glucose. Any glucose that is not used immediately for energy is changed into glycogen and stored in your liver and muscles to be used later. The glucose level in your blood then reduces to normal.

To maintain this balance in blood sugar, your body works in a similar way to the thermostat on a central heating system. Your natural 'thermostat' clicks into action as glucose levels rise and fall and your body will take action in the following ways.

When the glucose level falls too low:

The stress hormones adrenaline and cortisol are released from your adrenal glands and glucagon is produced by your pancreas. Glucagon is a pancreatic hormone that raises blood sugar. It works in the opposite way to insulin, encouraging your liver to turn some of its glycogen stores back into glucose, to give you a quick boost of energy. If your blood-glucose levels stay low for a period of time a state called hypoglycaemia – low blood sugar – can occur.

Symptoms of low blood sugar can include:

- irritability
- aggressive outbursts
- palpitations
- lack of sex drive
- crying spells
- dizziness
- anxiety
- confusion
- forgetfulness
- inability to concentrate
- fatigue
- insomnia
- headaches
- muscle cramps
- excess sweating
- excessive thirst

Chances are that if you have a history of dieting then some, many, or even all of these symptoms will be familiar. In themselves, they can be burdensome but, more importantly, they are the outward signs that your body is having trouble stabilising your blood sugar level. They're the flashing light on the heating system warning that something's wrong. They will, without doubt, undermine your diet plan by triggering unhealthy eating which, in turn, contributes to weight gain.

When the glucose level rises too high:

Insulin is produced by the pancreas to lower blood glucose (sugar). If the blood sugar level remains too high this causes symptoms of hyperglycaemia - high blood sugar.

Symptoms can include:

- frequent (often extreme) hunger and/or thirst
- frequent urination
- blurred vision
- fatigue
- dry or itchy skin
- cardiac arrhythmia (erratic heartbeat)
- poor wound healing

- dry mouth
- tingling in feet or heels
- frequent infections

Chronic and extreme hyperglycaemia can lead to insulin resistance (or 'pre-diabetes') and ultimately type 2 diabetes, a serious, lifelong medical condition. Weight cycling or yo-yoing – where you gain weight, lose it, gain it and so on – may make you more prone to type 2 diabetes. Being overweight in general is also a clear risk factor – the greater your weight, the higher your risk of developing type 2 diabetes.

How food and drink affects blood sugar

During a normal day, the amount by which your blood sugar level rises and falls depends on what and when you eat. When you eat any carbohydrates in a refined (processed) form, digestion happens very quickly. Refined foods have been stripped of their natural goodness by various manufacturing processes. Two of the most widely used refined foods are sugar and white flour.

When digestion occurs too quickly, glucose enters your bloodstream too rapidly. This also happens when you take in any food or drink that has a stimulant effect, such as caffeine or chocolate. This sharp, fast rise in blood glucose makes you feel momentarily good, but the 'high' quickly passes and you plummet to a lower point, feeling tired and drained. So what do you do? Chances are, you quickly look for another fix – another bar of chocolate, another cup of coffee (or both!) to give you a further boost.

This second boost will cause your blood sugar level to rise rapidly again, and so the vicious cycle is repeated. As your blood sugar levels go up and down, so too do your eating patterns, encouraging cravings for sweet foods and drinks.

Over time, this constant overstimulation can lead to one of two issues. First, although you can be producing a lot of insulin, your cells can become insulin resistant and so the insulin can't do its job of moving the glucose from your blood into your cells. Hence the glucose (sugar) levels in your blood stay high and this overstimulation exhausts the pancreas. Or, instead of producing too much insulin, your pancreas produces too little and, once again, too much glucose stays in your blood. Both scenarios can result in type 2 diabetes.

> The answer to all this is to switch your diet to natural wholefoods, which are unrefined and full of goodness.

We'll look further at how they can help maintain balanced blood sugar levels later in this chapter.

When you eat is as important as what you eat

Let's look back at that old adage of dieting – that we should eat three meals a day without snacking in between. Remember I said it was a total myth? Well, here's why.

If you have long gaps between meals, your blood glucose will drop to quite a low level. Hence you will feel that need for a quick boost: you'll find yourself craving a cup of tea and a biscuit or a coffee and cupcake. At the same time, your adrenal glands will make your liver release glucose stores.

This combination causes high levels of glucose in the blood which, again, calls on your pancreas to over-produce insulin in order to reduce them. The vicious cycle starts all over again and the adrenal glands become ever more exhausted.

But really it's a problem that can easily be solved. Try:

- **Grazing.** Develop a 'grazing' habit in your eating patterns, eating little but often. Leave behind that old, outdated and, frankly *wrong*, dieting philosophy of no food between meals.
- **Avoid skipped meals.** You probably thought that if you ate less by missing meals you would lose weight? Wrong. The resultant swings in blood sugar are setting you up to fail. They create a biological urge that must be satisfied. Even if you were strong enough to ignore the cravings, they're a message from your body and we shouldn't ignore our body's demands. Instead, learn to understand what your body really needs.

Make it easy for yourself. Truly, losing weight need not be difficult or painful. If you stop the behaviour that is causing the biological urges, then you won't be constantly at war with your own body.

The effects of adrenaline and cortisol

If blood sugar levels are frequently low and your system is regularly being asked to pump out the stress hormones adrenaline and cortisol, there is no doubt that your health will suffer. Adrenaline is the hormone most of us associate with stress – it is released for the classic 'fight or flight' response and its effect is very powerful. If you were threatened in the street, for example, or faced with any kind of physical danger your survival mechanisms would instantly step into action with the adrenal glands producing large amounts of adrenaline and cortisol.

The effects of these stress hormones are that:

- your heart speeds up

- your arteries tighten to raise blood pressure
- your liver releases emergency stores of glucose to give you energy
- your digestion shuts down because it is not necessary for immediate survival
- the clotting ability of your blood is increased in case you are injured and start to bleed

In other words, your body is on high alert, ready for fight or flight. You can run faster, fight back and generally react more quickly than normal. Unfortunately, when your blood sugar level drops during the day or night, some adrenaline is released automatically and your body experiences all the above sensations, albeit at a lower level, except that there is no outside stress requiring a response. When this happens repeatedly, you can experience all the health problems outlined under the hypoglycaemia section earlier in this chapter. It can also contribute to heart disease by increasing the risk of blood clotting and higher blood pressure and the sudden release of glucose for energy can cause extreme fluctuations of sugar levels in your blood.

These fluctuations in blood sugar create internal stress – and your body has to deal with it. Your digestive system will not function efficiently and less stomach acid will be produced, which means that food may not be digested sufficiently and will be stored for a longer time in your gut. The longer food stays in your intestines and remains undigested, the more calories are absorbed. (Digestion is a balancing game. It is important that food is moved quickly through your intestines, but not *so* quickly that valuable nutrients are not absorbed.) Along with all these changes, your body has to call on supplies of vitamins and minerals to deal with this internal stress. If you are continually stressed, your body becomes increasingly nutritionally deficient.

Cravings vs binges

Are you a craver or a binger? And does it make a difference to how you lose weight? Let's look at the difference. Remember, knowledge is power – the more you understand the way your body works, the more easily you will be able to work *with* your body, rather than against it. You will learn how to lose weight in harmony with your body, rather than constantly fighting against it.

Cravings: Most dieters experience cravings to a lesser or greater degree. For some it's sweet foods – chocolate, biscuits, cakes. Some people crave fats, like cream and hard cheese. Others yearn for savoury, salty snacks – crisps and crackers. Even if you're not a habitual drinker of alcohol, you might sometimes crave a glass of wine or a cold beer.

If you experience cravings, the likely explanation is blood sugar imbalance. Other cravings may have their origins in a food intolerance or perhaps a yeast problem – we will look at these factors in depth in Chapter 5.

By and large you can control your own cravings, even those linked to the hormonal ups and downs of the menstrual cycle. It might be hard at first but by following the rules in this chapter you will find it becomes easier with the passing of each successful day. Eventually the cravings will cease.

Bingeing: Bingeing can signal a more serious problem. Giving into a craving and eating a bar of chocolate or several biscuits is not bingeing. A binge is eating for eating's sake, almost uncontrollably and even when you aren't hungry. Bingers have been known to grab at food with their hands rather than waste time with a knife and fork. There is a desperation about bingers and many people who binge-eat often do so in response to an emotional upset. Eating non-stop until you've finished a family-size tub of ice cream, or a complete gateau, for example, is bingeing. So too is eating to the point of being sick. This is a long way from the normal cravings that most dieters experience.

Bingers will often feel physically and mentally ill after they've binged and binging can be associated with serious illnesses, such as bulimia. Bulimia is characterised by an insatiable desire for food, sometimes with episodes of continuous eating which is followed by purging and depression.

If you know that you binge, I would strongly advise that you seek help from your doctor in the first place. You really do need medical and psychological support to help you overcome this.

Beating the blood sugar rollercoaster

So, how can we prevent this constant cycle, this crazy rollercoaster of highs and lows? There are three simple ways:

1. Eat unrefined carbohydrates
2. Avoid refined carbohydrates, especially sugar
3. Reduce foods and drinks that are stimulants

Let's look at these in more detail.

1. Eat unrefined carbohydrates

Carbohydrates are a large group of foods that include sugar and starches. They are an important source of energy and your body breaks them down into glucose. It is the speed with which this happens that is important in keeping blood glucose (sugar) stable.

For me, the important issue about carbohydrates is that they need to be unrefined – in other words not processed but still close to their natural state. The more refined the carbohydrate, the more fibre has been removed, and the faster the hit on your bloodstream. This is because your body can break it down into glucose faster.

To maintain well-balanced blood sugar levels, you should eat foods containing unrefined carbohydrates. This will result in a slow, even rise in blood sugar that will remain constant for about three hours. After three hours, you will need to eat again to prevent the level from dropping. Spacing food at three-hourly intervals in this way is a proven solution to the battle with cravings. Simple? Yes, incredibly. But, truthfully, it works.

'Unrefined' means unprocessed – the food is closest to its natural state. So that means whole wheat pasta and bread (not white), brown rice, barley, millet, maize, oats, rye, spelt, amaranth. In contrast, refined carbohydrates have been processed – usually the outer layers of the grain have been removed, along with essential vitamins, minerals, trace elements and valuable fibre. Think white rice, white flour and all the products which are then made from refined white flour, such as pasta, bread, biscuits, cakes, pastry, pies and so on. In order to digest these refined foods your body has to use its own vitamins and minerals, so depleting your own stores.

With fruit, there is a big difference between eating an orange or drinking a glass of orange juice. There could be eight oranges in a glass of juice but you wouldn't sit down and eat eight oranges at one time. Because the fibre from the oranges has been removed, the juice is going to increase your blood glucose much more quickly than the whole fruit would.

To help you maintain a steady blood sugar level, aim to eat unrefined carbohydrates as part of your main meals and also as snacks during the day. You do not necessarily need to eat large amounts – sometimes just an oat cake can be enough between meals to keep eating urges at bay.

You may find that the symptoms associated with low blood sugar levels are strongest first thing in the morning (maybe you wake up with a headache or feel dizzy or weak), or you wake during the night with your heart pounding and cannot get back to sleep. If so, it is very likely that your blood sugar level has dropped overnight and adrenaline has kicked into play. Eating a small snack, like an oatcake, one hour before going to bed and, if possible, having breakfast within one hour of getting up will help to alleviate these symptoms.

Unrefined carbohydrates are also a great source of dietary fibre. It was originally thought that the only role of fibre in the diet was to speed up the passage of food residues through the intestines and hence prevent constipation. This is an important role and should not be dismissed – as we have already discussed, the longer food stays in your body, the more calories it absorbs and the harder it is to shed those pounds/kilos. However, the role of fibre is more complex than that and we now know that some forms of fibre can actually slow down the absorption of sugars and help to maintain your blood sugar balance.

2. Avoid refined carbohydrates, especially sugar

Avoid all refined carbohydrates where possible. This includes all the white foods mentioned above and all the processed sweeteners that can be added to foods such as sugar (sucrose), dextrose, maltose, fructose, corn syrup. I have covered some of these sweeteners in more detail on page 81.

As mentioned above, be careful of fruit juices – they count as refined because the fibre has been removed. A smoothie is better because it blends the food without removing fibre. It will still be absorbed faster than the whole fruit because it is a liquid, but slower than the fruit juice. You could add vegetables to the smoothie, which will slow the absorption further and also some protein like cashew nuts.

If you start looking at labels, you will be amazed at how sugar sneaks unexpectedly into a vast number of foods.

When it comes to sugar, I'm afraid we can't follow the 'brown is best' rule. Every colour of sugar does the same damage to your blood sugar balance (and also to your body in general). White table sugar is the same as soft brown sugar, as demerara, as golden syrup... A can of cola may contain up to 120ml (eight whole teaspoons) of added sugar. So too can a pot of fruit yogurt (and that's not even counting the sugar naturally contained in the fruit). Most of the convenience foods and drinks we buy are laden with sugar – not just the sweet ones but also some savoury foods such as baked beans and mayonnaise. Did you know that tomato ketchup has just eight per cent less sugar, weight for weight, than ice cream and that the cream substitute for coffee is 65 per cent sugar compared to 51 per cent for a chocolate bar?

It is estimated that, even if you don't add sugar to your tea and coffee, you can be consuming around 46 teaspoons of sugar every day simply because it is added (and hidden) in so many foods (both sweet and savoury).

You may be tempted to substitute sugar with artificial sweeteners – **DON'T!** You will simply be introducing a foreign chemical which your body then has to deal with. Many diet gurus and plans rely heavily on sugar substitutes and artificial sweeteners to avoid calorific sugar. I strongly disagree with this strategy. Studies have clearly shown that they confuse your body and don't help you lose weight. In fact, they can *increase* your appetite and make you gain weight[31].

How? Normally when you taste something sweet it comes with a chunk of calories that pacify the body. But artificial sweeteners have no calories so your body sends you off to find those calories somewhere else and it does this by increasing your appetite and giving you cravings.

When rats are fed artificial sweeteners they take in more calories, weigh more and, even more worryingly, this weight is made up of an increase in body fat percentage. The artificial sweeteners change the animals' inner control of knowing when they have had enough to eat[32].

Research has shown that people who drink two or more diet drinks a day have waist circumference increases 500 per cent greater than people who don't drink diet drinks[33]. And they can increase your risk of type 2 diabetes and cardiovascular disease[34]. If any food or drink is described as 'low sugar', 'no-sugar' or 'diet' it will nearly always contain an artificial sweetener. These chemical sweeteners can also be found in 'non-diet' foods and drinks and also in some medications. It's worth checking labels carefully. Over the course of a day you may be taking in several foods and drinks containing artificial sweeteners – these will band together to produce a cumulative effect. If you take a variety of different sweeteners you will be giving your body a veritable cocktail of nasties as the various chemicals combine. This will have a further (highly detrimental) effect on your body. We will be looking at artificial sweetness and label reading in more depth in chapter 4. For now, start becoming label aware, and start dropping unrefined carbohydrates from your diet.

3. Reduce foods and drinks that are stimulants

We love stimulants – we adore the wide-awake buzz they give us. Whether it's a sugary snack, a comforting bar of chocolate, the caffeine shot from coffee, tea, hot chocolate or soft drinks or the nicotine hit from tobacco, stimulants make us feel good. But only in the short term. Stimulants cause a fast rise in blood sugar level followed by a quick drop which contributes to the rollercoaster ride of blood sugar swings. It can sound like a tough call to avoid them entirely but, trust me, your body will love you for it – and your mind will also have the chance to become naturally alert and well-balanced.

Hot stimulant drinks are so ingrained in our culture, it can be tough to let them go, but try substituting them with, for example, herbal teas, chicory or grain coffee alternatives, turmeric lattes, diluted pure fruit and vegetable juices and, of course, pure filtered water. Don't just switch to decaffeinated coffee, tea or colas. It may seem a good idea but they contain other stimulants even when the caffeine is removed.

Be careful to come off these stimulants slowly, or you may have temporary withdrawal issues like headaches and flu-like symptoms. Better to switch half your drinks to caffeinated, then reduce by one more drink a day for the next few days. Remember to replace them with non-stimulant alternatives, so you're still having the same fluid intake.

• In summary: your at-a-glance guide to balancing your blood sugar •

DO

- Eat unrefined carbohydrates including: brown rice, millet, oats, rye, spelt and wholewheat.
- Eat fruit.
- Always eat breakfast.
- Eat small, frequent meals, no more than three hours apart.
- Reduce, and preferably avoid, stimulants including tea, coffee, chocolate, soft drinks and sodas (all contain sugar or artificial sweeteners and many also contain caffeine) and tobacco.
- Consider taking a good supplement programme that can balance your blood sugar while you are changing your eating patterns. This will be explained fully in Chapter 7.
- Develop the habit of reading labels carefully.

DON'T

- Eat refined carbohydrates – avoid 'white' things in general. White flour is in nearly all processed foods, in particular cakes, biscuits, pastries, pasta and white bread.
- Eat sugar or foods or drinks containing sugar – including chocolate, sweets, biscuits, pastries, fruit yogurts, soft drinks, many savoury foods like tomato sauces, ketchup and so on. Check all labels.
- Substitute artificial sweeteners or decaffeinated drinks.
- Eat convenience foods as they are likely to contain refined carbohydrates, sugar and high levels of fat and salt.

Glycaemic Index and Glycaemic Load

Using the Glycaemic Index (GI) to help weight control has been gaining in popularity over the last few years. As it has an important impact on blood sugar balance, it's something well worth taking the time to understand.

As I've already mentioned, some carbohydrates have a 'fast-releasing' effect while others are 'slow-releasing' and it has been found that this releasing effect can be measured against glucose. This method of measuring has become known as the Glycaemic Index (GI). As glucose is the fastest-releasing carbohydrate, and raises insulin to the highest level, the index gives glucose a score of 100 – everything else is measured against this score.

Raised insulin levels encourage fat to be stored in your body. But if you have high insulin levels because your blood sugar keeps fluctuating, you will not only change more of your food into fat, you will also prevent your body breaking down previously stored fat. It's a bit like adding money to your bank account without spending any. That's fine with cash but not so good when it comes to fat. No wonder they are called 'fat deposits'.

This is why it's so incredibly important to follow the recommendations given in the first half of this chapter. These will optimise and balance insulin levels, keeping fat storage to a minimum. Whole foods, such as brown rice, are important because the fibre these foods contain slows down the release of sugars and gives them a lower GI. The same goes for fruit rather than fruit juice because of the fibre content of the fruit.

Adding protein to the mix

We've already learned how important unrefined carbohydrates are if we want to keep blood sugar levels balanced and hence encourage our bodies to lose weight. GI adds another important factor – it is highly beneficial to combine unrefined carbohydrates with protein at the same meal.

The idea of combining carbohydrates and protein has been practiced for centuries in traditional cultures where a meal will automatically contain foods such as lentils and rice. The Japanese, for example, often have rice, fish, and soya at each meal, along with vegetables. It was virtually unheard of to see an overweight Japanese person until the introduction of a Western diet in Japan.

The presence of protein in food (either animal or vegetable, like tofu) actually lowers its GI. So pulses, such as lentils, which naturally contain both protein and carbohydrate, have a low GI.

This flies directly in the face of food combining (or rather not combining) which, we saw in the last chapter, advocates keeping protein and carbohydrate strictly apart. While there is a place for food combining (it can be helpful for some digestive problems), it can make matters much worse for those with blood sugar imbalances. Of course, we are all individuals, so it is important to keep in mind your own circumstances. If your case is complicated, it may also be worth coming to one of my Glenville Nutrition Clinics (see Resources Page 158).

There are many GI charts available in books and online but, unfortunately, they are not very helpful because the GI of a food can change depending on a number of factors including:

- The ripeness of the food – riper yellow bananas have a higher GI than green ones
- The physical form of the food (its particle size – mashing a one inch cube of potato increases its GI by 25 per cent)
- Variability within food classes:
    1. Type (different shapes of pasta, for instance)
    2. Processing (grinding and pressing can increase the GI)
    3. Preparation (cooking increases GI)

Refining GI – Glycaemic Load

The other problem with the GI index is that it can be hugely confusing. For example, on many charts you will see that chocolate has a lower GI than watermelon (48 compared to 72 for watermelon). This is because the GI doesn't tell you how much carbohydrate the food contains. So you'd have to eat a huge amount of watermelon (because of its low carbohydrate content) compared to the small amount of chocolate you can eat to get the same change in blood sugar. Carrots on the GI charts also have the same GI as chocolate.

The answer to this problem comes with another measure – the Glycaemic Load. This calculates how much carbohydrate there is in the food. So the effect on your blood sugar is determined, not only by the quality of the carbohydrate (GI) but by the quantity (GL).

So, let's look at that watermelon again. It contains 6gms of carbohydrate per 100gms and the GL is calculated by:

GL = 72 (the GI of watermelon) x 6gms of carbohydrate = 43.2 divided by 100gms = 4.32

So the GL is only 4.32 compared to 14 for chocolate.

How does the Glycaemic Index/Load work in everyday life?

Research has shown that obese people who eat even *unlimited* quantities of low GI foods lose more weight than obese people on a low fat, low calorie diet[35]. So yes it does work. Yet, as fascinating as the GI and GL are, I don't think it is a good idea to swap one set of restrictive numbers for another. Having persuaded you to stop thinking about calories, the last thing I want is for you to start obsessing about GI and GL.

The easiest way to think about it all is this: if the food is refined (stripped of fibre) then it is going to hit your blood stream faster and the higher your blood sugar will rise in response to it. The consequence of this will be that your pancreas will produce more insulin to deal with it and, the bottom line, insulin is your fat storing hormone.

So, when you eat an unrefined carbohydrate, do have some protein with it (either animal or vegetable based) as this automatically lowers the GI response, slowing down the rate at which the food gets digested. For example, think about a little hummus, cheese or nut butter on your oatcake, or some nuts and seeds and natural yogurt on your wholegrain muesli. Drizzling oil on a starchy carbohydrate can also lower the GI, as can adding vinegar or lemon juice (by as much as 20-40 per cent). Vinegar is also thought to slow down the rate at which food leaves your stomach.

Using the power of your mind to help food cravings

As we've discovered, most of the problems with cravings come about purely through your body's biochemistry. If you take away the rollercoaster of blood sugar surges, you will automatically eliminate most cravings. However, it's important to note that we are emotional beings and that our thoughts and emotions are also a factor in weight loss. Let's look at a few psychological tips to help gain control over food cravings.

1. Know your triggers

Become aware of when you crave certain foods. Keep a food diary and identify situations that cause you to overeat. If you know that certain situations make you feel the need for certain foods, either avoid them or prepare yourself by taking something else to eat that may satisfy that need in a more healthy manner. So, for example, if you work in a place where everyone brings in cakes and sugary snacks to share, prepare yourself with tasty low GI snacks.

2. Ask yourself if your emotions are a trigger?

Do you eat differently when you feel sad, lonely, stressed or bored? We know that stress can play a large part in weight control. Research has shown that if you sit two groups of people (dieters and non-dieters) in front of a stressful film and give them peanuts and chocolates, the non-dieters will nibble absent-mindedly but the dieters can eat three times the quantity of food during the film[36].

Look at what else you could substitute in place of food. Fill your life with other things which will keep you active, keep your mind off the subject of food and help keep negative feelings at bay. Find a new hobby, perhaps one you enjoy doing at home, especially in the evenings, like knitting, sewing or reading. Join an evening class – there are endless options. You could learn a new language, a new skill, or take up a new sport.

3. Become aware of habit eating

It is very easy to get into habits such as eating while driving or eating while watching TV or at the cinema. These can become so ingrained that you end up always associating food with specific activities. Eating while busily doing something else is a dangerous combination because you become unaware of the quantities you are eating. Separate out eating from other activities. Become very aware when you eat and eat mindfully, keeping your entire focus on your food. Break the association of this unconscious eating. At first it may feel difficult, particularly if you're used to snacking in the evening while watching TV. Try doing something to occupy your hands, such as sewing, knitting, even painting your nails.

Have a look at what has become automatic. Do you always buy something to eat on the way home from work or go straight to the fridge when you get in? Again, this action can be almost unconscious. A vital key is to become aware of what you are doing and when. Stop, think and ask yourself: 'Do I really need to eat this now? Will I be happy with the way I feel after I have eaten it?'

Ask yourself if you are actually hungry, or could you in fact be thirsty? Sometimes these messages get confused and we are really feeling dehydrated rather than hungry. Try drinking a glass of water, then see if you still feel hungry. Enjoy your food. If you decide to eat a bar of chocolate then fine, but just eat the bar of chocolate. Don't watch TV or read the newspaper while you do it. Really taste the chocolate, eating it really slowly and mindfully, being fully aware of the textures and flavours. Don't feel guilty about eating it – just make sure you really enjoy every single nibble.

4. Get some exercise

Exercise releases chemicals called endorphins that make you feel good. Going for a brisk walk or a swim when you feel cravings can even ward off the urge to binge. The exercise will also suppress your appetite for a while afterwards. If you tend to eat when you are angry or stressed, try going for a vigorous walk, cycle or run as soon as negative feelings strike. I'll look at exercise more in Chapter 6.

5. Distract yourself

Cravings will subside even if you don't satisfy them. Do something else – read, make a phone call, get that household chore done – and see how you feel after that.

6. Don't deny yourself

If you say to yourself you are never going to eat chocolate again, you will almost certainly fail. Be realistic. We are all going to eat foods that we are really better off without. If the main foundations of your diet are good, relax. Go away on holiday and enjoy yourself. If you are out with friends for a treat, don't deny yourself if they are eating pizza or ice-cream. If you keep denying yourself you will develop problems of self-denial and the craving may just reach explosion point with you eating far more than if you had allowed yourself a small treat now and again. But, really, this shouldn't be a problem if you follow the guidelines in this book. If you eat little and often, focusing on good unrefined carbohydrates (with a little protein), you will find your cravings automatically subside.

Case history

Mary came to me with digestive problems and a feeling of being constantly tired. She had a lot of flatulence and felt bloated after each meal, saying it felt as though she were 'eight months pregnant'. She also mentioned having sugar cravings which were 'stronger than those for cigarettes'.

I put her on a good supplement programme including chromium (see Chapter 7) and we talked about blood sugar swings and the need to eat little and often with more emphasis on eating unrefined carbohydrates.

At her follow-up consultation Mary said that she now 'believed in miracles'. She was sleeping more soundly, her digestion was better and she was eating more regularly. She particularly noticed a difference in her energy levels.

A letter she sent later said: 'I'm happy to report that I have felt very much more energetic. So much so that a couple of people have commented on my jaunty behaviour.'

The mood and food connection – why chocolate is a comfort food

There's a reason chocolate is a go-to for many of us when we feel down. It contains substances that produce the same feelgood buzz we get when we're in love. In fact, research has shown that the chemicals in chocolate target the same brain receptors as marijuana.

Scientists have now found that foods can trigger important changes in our brain chemistry. What we eat and drink can determine whether we feel happy or depressed. These powerful brain chemicals can also affect our appetite and our ability to control it.

Brain chemicals

Within your brain there are chemicals known as neurotransmitters which transmit signals to neurones (brain cells). Some of these brain chemicals can control your appetite which is vital for you to survive. We need to feel hungry to keep us alive and yet we also need to feel satisfied to know when to stop eating.

These brain chemicals *increase* your intake of food:

- endorphins
- norepinephrine (noradrenaline)
- neuropeptide Y

These *decrease* your intake of food:

- cholecystokinin (CCK)
- serotonin
- corticotropin releasing factor

How do these brain chemicals make you feel?

- Serotonin makes us feel calm and can lift depression
- Norepinephrine (noradrenaline) makes us feel alert and energetic
- Endorphins can give a 'natural buzz' – a sense of euphoria

Carbohydrates increase the levels of serotonin, which controls your appetite and makes you feel good. A higher-carbohydrate meal causes a larger proportion of tryptophan, an amino acid, to get to your brain in order to stimulate the production of serotonin.

Carbohydrates help your body to release insulin, and this increases the uptake of the other amino acids, leaving the tryptophan to dominate. On the other hand, when we eat a protein heavy meal or snack, a number of amino acids including tryptophan are competing to get into the brain and therefore the tryptophan cannot dominate.

Therefore carbohydrates make you feel happier and more relaxed and control your appetite for the next meal. Eating little and often and keeping your blood sugar in balance means that you can control your moods and also your appetite without feeling deprived or hungry. If you eat too little, your serotonin level, which regulates mood and appetite, will fall and then you will start to overeat.

Protein contains an amino acid called tyrosine which manufactures the neurotransmitters norepinephrine (noradrenaline) and dopamine which help to focus your mind and keep you alert.

Hunger hormones

It's not just these neurotransmitters that affect your appetite. Remember those hormones that make you feel hungry or satisfied: ghrelin and leptin?

There should be a fine balance of eating when you are hungry and stopping when you are full. But if you are overweight the system falls down and your brain can end up getting the wrong signals. A person who is overweight has more fat cells and so more leptin is produced. At first sight, this would seem to be a good thing as leptin reduces hunger but, as with insulin, over time your body can become leptin resistant. So the leptin level in the body may be high but your body will not be registering it. Your brain is simply not getting the message that you are full. All it hears is that you are hungry.

But how can we apply this knowledge to weight loss? Well, understanding the different biochemical reactions of food on your mood means you can use it to your advantage and eat the right foods at the right time. Let's look at a typical day:

Breakfast - Having a mainly carbohydrate breakfast, such as porridge oats, has a positive mood-enhancing effect. Add in some protein via ground nuts and seeds to make the energy release even more slow-releasing – perfect for balancing blood sugar levels. It is important to eat breakfast, but if you find this makes you feel hungrier during the day (as some of my clients have said), try eating a mainly protein breakfast, such as scrambled eggs, with a slice of wholemeal or rye bread. Both unrefined carbohydrates and protein reduce levels of the hunger hormone ghrelin.

Lunch – In order to feel alert and focused in the afternoon, eat a predominantly protein meal for lunch such as a tuna salad with a small portion of brown rice or a rye cracker. If you have a mainly carbohydrate meal, such as a jacket potato, it can make you feel relaxed and sleepy. Your body naturally has a 'post lunch dip' in the afternoon and a carbohydrate meal at lunch will promote this. Many countries enjoy a siesta after lunch but such luxuries don't fit into everyone's working day and, if affected, we have to battle our way through the dreaded afternoon slump.

Dinner – If you are turning to alcohol to help you relax in the evening, try skipping the wine and having a higher carbohydrate evening meal such as rice and tofu stir-fry or rice and fish – the starchy carbohydrate can help relax you instead of the alcohol. If alcohol is *not* an issue for you, you will lose weight faster if you cut down the starchy carbohydrates at your evening meal, and choose protein (fish, eggs, tofu) combined with vegetables and salad. You can always use quinoa, which is a seed and not a grain, instead of the starchy carbohydrate as it will seem like you are eating rice but it is actually a protein.

Snacks – Remember to eat something every three hours. So factor in snacks mid-morning and mid-afternoon to avoid blood sugar slumps. And try and include a protein with a carbohydrate such as apple with nuts or seeds, oatcakes with nut butter, crudités with hummus.

These are purely suggestions. We are all so different, so take the time to look at your own daily pattern and work out what different kinds of food are appropriate, and at which times, for you. Keeping a food diary will help you notice which foods have which effect on your energy and mood, and allow you to adjust your choices.

Other ways of controlling your appetite

1. *Eat more slowly.* This allows your brain, and in turn your appetite, time to receive the signals that you have eaten enough. The chemical cholecystokinin (CCK) is released as food enters your stomach. It tells your digestion to slow down and then gives the message to your brain that you are 'full' and your appetite naturally decreases. This message takes time – about 20 minutes.

2. *Exercise.* Research has shown that exercise decreases the feelings of hunger and causes the level of ghrelin (the hormone that stimulates your appetite) to drop[37].

3. *Sleep.* It's vital that you get enough sleep. If you are sleep deprived, this can increase your appetite. If you don't get a good amount of sleep (six to eight hours a night is ideal), your hunger hormone ghrelin is over-produced and leptin levels, which suppress your appetite, are decreased. A large study of nearly 70,000 women conducted over 16 years found that those who slept less than five hours a night gained more weight over time than those who slept for 7 hours a night[38].

4. *Eat a wide and varied diet.* The balance of your brain chemicals can be disturbed by nutritional deficiencies and by poor diet. The more restricted your choice of foods, the harder it is for your body to help your brain to maintain this important balance of neurotransmitters.

• Chapter 3 •

A Way of Life – Not a Diet

It may already have dawned on you that this book isn't just about losing weight. In fact, losing weight is merely a by-product of the plan. The way of eating I advocate is not a diet – it's a plan for life. It's all about giving your body the exact food it needs so you can not only look good but feel fantastic. This way of eating offers you total health and wellbeing, naturally.

As you've already seen, it's all about working *with* your body, providing it with the exact fuel it needs to work at its best. It works because it's natural, it's sustainable, and it's delicious.

In contrast, the majority of diets work *against* your body, demanding it functions unnaturally, giving it unnatural foods and substances that confuse and alarm it.

Really, it's simple. We are natural beings and the fuel our bodies require is exactly that – *natural*. Untampered with, unrefined, uncomplicated, simple.

Your body knows exactly what to do with natural foods. It can digest them easily and use them to its maximum benefit. These are the foods you can burn off swiftly, which means they are good suppliers of energy and don't linger in your body causing weight gain.

Make a shift to eating for life, rather than eating to diet, and your body will thank you. It will show its appreciation by returning to your optimum weight. It will also make you feel wonderfully healthy – with more energy, vitality, clarity of mind and general *joie de vivre*.

Research by scientists worldwide is now showing that if you look after yourself you have a better chance of preventing certain degenerative illnesses such as heart disease, type 2 diabetes and cancer, including breast and bowel cancer[39].

As an analogy, if you put poor-quality petrol into a high performance car it may run for a while but eventually it will become less efficient and the engine will deteriorate. It is exactly the same with the human body. You need top-grade fuel to run on all cylinders. Survival is your body's top priority and it will use whatever nourishment you give it to stay alive. Providing it with a quality diet will naturally ease the body's task to keep you healthy and it will also help you maintain a comfortable weight.

The eating plan outlined in this chapter is an enjoyable, pleasurable and healthy way of eating. It won't give you the very quick, early weight loss that you experience with so many diets – but that's a *good* thing. For safe, sustainable weight loss, you need to lose slowly, gradually, carefully. No more than two pounds a week. It might not sound a lot but week-on-week it soon adds up to a new you and, most importantly, it lasts.

Let me be very clear. This is not a way of eating that you follow for a short while and then abandon and go back to your former unhealthy eating patterns. The idea is that you embrace a whole new concept of nourishing yourself that is full of variety and taste. By eliminating foods that are not good for you and concentrating on foods that are healthy, you will find this becomes a way of life that is easy to follow – I promise you won't feel deprived.

The 80/20 Rule

There may be occasions when it is not possible to follow the guidelines exactly, perhaps when you are being entertained by others. So long as you have a foundation of eating well, then the odd deviation will not matter. Think of the 80/20 rule. This states that, providing you eat well for 80 per cent of the time, the occasional lapses for birthdays, holidays and parties won't hurt. Aiming for 100 per cent is setting yourself up for a tough time. You're only human, so give yourself a break. By using the 80/20 rule, you will simply shrug aside the 'naughty' 20 per cent and focus on making the vast majority of your food health-giving and kind to your body.

Above all, food is to be enjoyed. Eating is a time for sharing and socialising. There is nothing more demoralising than turning down invites to eat with friends because you are frightened you will slip from your diet.

Gradually change your eating habits

Some small changes that will make your eating healthy are fairly easy to adopt – such as drinking sparkling water with a slice of lemon instead of squash or fizzy sodas. Others may be harder, such as giving up coffee, tea and sugary snacks. Don't be discouraged because you think that altering your eating habits sounds too difficult. Try taking it one step at a time. You'll be pleasantly surprised at how well you can adapt to changes if they're gradual. Once you start to feel and see the benefits, you'll know that it was all worthwhile.

I truly believe that knowledge is power and once you understand how food and drinks affect your body, it becomes much easier to make informed choices. You can take control of your weight and health.

You are what you eat

All the food and drink that goes through your mouth has an effect on your body and mind. It will strengthen or weaken you; help or hinder; nourish or deplete. Food need not be your enemy – in the right form it's a valuable friend.

The physiological functions described in this book can be quite technical but are explained here in simple terms.

The human body is comprised of approximately 62 per cent water, 16 per cent protein, 16 per cent fat, six per cent minerals, less than one per cent carbohydrate and a small amount of vitamins. A woman's body carries more fat percentage than men so the other amounts will vary slightly.

Water is an essential nutrient that is involved in every function of your body. It helps transport nutrients and waste products in and out of your cells.

Protein is the basic building block for all your cells and bones as well as your hair, skin and nails. It is made up from 25 amino acids, eight of which are called 'essential' because you must get them from your diet. The other 17 can be made by your own body. To make sure you are getting the 'essential' eight it is vital to eat good-quality, protein-rich foods including eggs, fish, pulses, nuts and seeds.

Fat is important. We demonise it unfairly. Fat keeps you warm, insulates your nerve cells, feeds your brain and is a component of every human cell. Some fats are essential (as with the amino acids we have to take them in from our diet or as supplements) while others aren't. We will look at the difference later in this chapter.

Minerals are a natural part of your make-up and are vital for your survival.

While protein and fat are important, the primary source of energy that keeps all this functioning properly and gives you energy for living is carbohydrates which come from grains (rice, wheat, oats, corn), fruits and vegetables.

• Optional Extra: the 12-hour eating window •

Remember back in Chapter 1 we talked about intermittent fasting? I'm not a fan of extreme versions, but it is a way of eating (not a diet!) that offers health benefits. If you want to give it a try, I would suggest the 12:12 plan. That means you eat within a 12 hour window, then not for the next 12 hours. For example you finish eating for the evening by 8pm and then don't have anything until breakfast at 8am, or 7pm to 7am, 6pm to 6am – whatever works for you.

It has been suggested that restricting food intake to 12 hours a day prevents excessive weight gain, improves sleep and reduces age- and diet-related heart deterioration[40].

When overweight people who normally ate during a greater than 14-hour window were asked to eat only during a maximum of a 12-hour window for 16 weeks, they lost weight, had more energy and slept better and these benefits lasted for a year[41].

This isn't a compulsory part of my plan, but I suggest it as I think you might feel the benefits if you decide to give it a go.

Steps toward a new way of eating

Even accounting for personal preference and different lifestyles there are certain steps we can *all* take to improve our health and maintain a healthy weight.

1. Eat unrefined carbohydrates.
2. Stabilise your blood sugar levels by reducing your intake of refined foods.
3. Reduce tea, coffee and alcohol – they contribute to the problem of blood sugar imbalances and can deprive your body of vital nutrients and trace elements.
4. Reduce your intake of dairy products.
5. Reconsider meat and poultry.
6. Know your fats.
7. Increase your natural fibre intake.
8. Reduce salt in your diet.

Let's look at each of these areas in more detail.

1. Eat unrefined carbohydrates

The benefits from eating unrefined carbohydrates are discussed fully in Chapter 2 – they give us the sustained energy and fibre we need for good health.

2. Stabilise blood sugar levels

This is vital to successful weight loss as we have already discussed in Chapter 2. Remember how blood sugar dips lead to cravings? Even if you don't have a problem with cravings, it's important to stick to the general guidelines to avoid fluctuations in blood sugar levels. The more you know about how your body's biochemistry works, the easier it is to make good choices and to reach your ideal weight.

3. Avoid addictive drinks

Alcohol, tea, coffee and colas (either diet or regular) are socially acceptable drugs and they have either a depressant or a stimulant effect. Because they are part of everyday life we tend to forget their addictive properties. When we are younger, we are adaptable, flexible and able to eliminate toxins with ease. As we get older our bodies have less tolerance and the effects accumulate. Behaviour we could get away with as teenagers unfortunately catches up with us as we move into our 30s, 40s and beyond. As our bodies become less efficient we end up storing too much of what we don't actually need.

Coffee

Coffee contains three stimulants – caffeine, theobromine and theophylline. A cup of instant coffee (8oz) contains around 66mg of caffeine; filtered coffee contains 120mg and even decaffeinated coffee still contains 5mg.

As outlined in Chapter 2, the stimulant effect of caffeine is often quickly followed by a 'downer' which encourages you to have another cup and so the cycle is born. Also the diuretic effect of caffeine may flush vital nutrients and trace elements out of your body.

Another problem with coffee is that the active ingredients in caffeine (called methylxanthines) have been linked to a benign breast disease known as fibrocystic disease. Many women experience breast discomfort in the week before a period that can become worse and develop into mastalgia (breast pain). The pain can be very intense and can occur at any time of the month. Many women have found relief from mastalgia purely by cutting out coffee. Methylxanthines are found in not only coffee but also chocolate, some canned drinks, cocoa and tea.

Stick to non-stimulant drinks like water, herbal teas or grain coffees.

Tea

Tea contains both caffeine and tannin. An 8oz cup of tea contains less caffeine than coffee - about 60mg – but the above effects of caffeine still apply and of course will depend on how much tea you drink a day. Green tea contains about 15mg caffeine per cup.

Tannin will make your teeth go brown, if you guzzle enough. It also binds important minerals such as iron, preventing their absorption in the digestive tract. If you must drink tea, don't have it with a meal because the vital nutrients from that meal will be wasted as they can be excreted unabsorbed.

So, are decaffeinated teas and coffees the answer? As I've suggested already, sadly not. Although decaffeinated coffee only contains a small amount of caffeine per cup (5mg), it still contains theobromine and theophylline, two chemicals that can disturb normal sleep patterns. Also decaffeinated coffee still contains the methylxanthines which, as we've seen, can cause breast problems. In addition, many decaffeinated coffees have been decaffeinated by chemical solvents such as methylene chloride or ethyl acetate. You can get coffee which has been decaffeinated by the Swiss Water Method and this is how organic coffee is decaffeinated as only water is used to eliminate the caffeine rather than chemicals.

Unlike coffee, when tea is decaffeinated, no other stimulants are left.

Coming off caffeine

Thankfully, more and more people are now becoming aware of the health problems associated with addictive drinks and are turning to alternatives. However, as with all drugs there can be quite dramatic withdrawal symptoms if you stop drinking caffeine too suddenly. These include:

- headaches
- nausea
- tiredness
- depression
- muscle pains
- flu-like symptoms

Some hospitals have now discovered that certain post-operative symptoms are not caused by the effects of the anaesthetic as previously thought, but by unintentional caffeine withdrawal. Before a general anaesthetic, patients are asked not to eat or drink for a number of hours and by the time they come round from the operation the withdrawal symptoms may have already started.

If you decide to cut caffeine from your daily routine, minimise these possible side effects by cutting down slowly over a period of a few weeks. Gradually substitute some of your usual caffeinated drinks for more healthy alternatives such as herbal teas, turmeric lattes and grain coffee (made with chicory). Do read the ingredients on these alternatives as some can contain added sugar.

Case history

Kate came to see me at my clinic with a long history of anxiety. For a number of years she had been on and off anti-depressants and felt she was in a downward spiral with mood swings, depression, dizziness and attacks of paranoia. She was also spotting from mid-cycle until her period arrived.

Her GP told her she was depressed and her gynaecologist advised her that her symptoms were caused by lack of oestrogen. She wanted to try for a child but said she couldn't imagine ever feeling well enough. I looked at Kate's questionnaire (all my patients fill in a questionnaire before a consultation) which showed that she was drinking six cups of tea plus some coffee every day, and was eating four or five biscuits and also cake on top of her regular meals. I talked about the effects of tea and coffee and the possible link between what she was eating and drinking and how she was feeling.

Kate stopped drinking tea and coffee and got headaches for three days while her body adjusted. She also took my advice and changed her eating pattern. Her anxiety and mood swings disappeared entirely. What amazed her most was the difference in other aspects of her health too. For the first time in three and a half years she had no spotting before her period. She had also been going regularly to the toilet each morning, which she hadn't done for 10 years as she had been suffering from constipation. She felt so much better that she decided to try for a baby.

Alcohol

Consumption of alcohol, especially wine, has been rising steadily in the UK. Most alcoholic drinks are made by the action of yeast on sugar, providing calories in the form of carbohydrates. One glass of wine provides us with 100 calories and a pint of beer with around 200 calories.

Not only does alcohol contribute to blood sugar imbalance but excessive drinking can also cause liver damage. Furthermore, it acts as an anti-nutrient – in other words it blocks the beneficial effects of our food by depleting vitamins and minerals, especially zinc. It also interferes with the metabolism of essential fatty acids which are so important for heart health, brain function, immune system and moods.

But what about the 'French paradox'? The French consume at least the same amount of saturated fat as we do and possibly more, and yet their rate of heart disease is much lower than in the UK. It was originally thought that wine, especially red wine, was protecting the French from heart problems, but now it seems that the protection is not from the alcohol in the wine but the actual grapes from which the wine is made. Grapes contain over 1600 beneficial compounds including important antioxidant polyphenols like resveratrol, catechins, anthocyanins, and flavonols[42]. The resveratrol is of most interest as it's been shown in studies to reduce cholesterol levels[43]. A glass of red wine contains approximately 100mg polyphenol, whereas grapes contain up to 300mg per 100g[44]. So save alcohol for special occasions and eat more grapes!

4. Reduce your intake of dairy products

Dairy products such as cheese, milk and cream should be used sparingly as they contain the protein casein. Casein is 300 times higher in cow's milk than it is in human milk so many people find that dairy products can be hard to digest.

Dairy products also contain lactose (milk sugar) and before this can be absorbed into the bloodstream from your gut it has to be broken down by the enzyme lactase into two other sugars, glucose and galactose. If you don't have enough lactase in your body then the lactose remains undigested in the gut and ferments, giving symptoms such as diarrhoea, abdominal pain, gas and bloating.

Milk has a low GI, which means that, in theory, it should not cause blood sugar fluctuations. But research has shown that it can cause a high level of insulin to be secreted[45]. If you add just 200ml milk to a low GI meal it causes an increase in insulin response by 300 per cent, thereby transforming it into a very high GI meal[46].

If you do wish to include dairy in your eating plan then choose organic plain live yogurt. This contains beneficial bacteria which are the natural inhabitants of your digestive system. Beware of fruit yogurts though as these can contain up to eight teaspoons of added sugar.

5. Reconsider meat and poultry

Protein is necessary for the structural formation of our bones, skin, hair and muscle and for healthy brain function. It is important, however, to monitor our intake of protein to ensure that not only are we getting a healthy amount, but that it is also coming from the healthiest sources. Excess protein has been linked to kidney stones, gout and high blood pressure.

The World Cancer Research Fund (WCRF) has stated that there is strong evidence linking red meat to bowel cancer. WCRF says that it is better to eat no more than 500g (cooked weight, about 700g raw weight) of red meat per week and to eliminate completely processed meats such as ham, bacon, salami, hot dogs and some sausages. Personally, I avoid red meat completely as there are other, healthier sources of animal protein, including fish and eggs. If you are going to eat red meat, then buy organic and, ideally, grass fed. (If meat is corn fed rather than grass fed, it will have higher amounts of omega 6 in its fat, which can contribute to inflammation in your body.)

Chicken and other poultry is often thought of as a healthier choice than red meat but in fact it can be pumped full of chemicals and water. Some chicken only contains about 51 per cent meat. Stabilisers, salt, lactose, glucose and dextrose can be used to hold water and offset the salt so the chicken looks plump and fresh. Flavour enhancers can also be used. If you are going to eat poultry then make sure it's organic. If cost is an issue then think quality rather than quantity and have it less often. Moving towards a more plant-based diet is better for your health and the environment.

6. Know your fats

The important point about fats is that some are essential and good for you and some are definitely not. Unfortunately, the bad name that fat has gained for itself over the years has unfairly affected the whole family of fats, with the result that too many people are trying to cut it out altogether.

As we've already seen, there are many low-fat and no-fat diets out there, both of which can be dangerous. Your body's only source of essential fats is from your diet (or supplements), so to cut out all fat is not sensible. Indeed fat-free diets can result in joint stiffness and skin problems as your body needs the lubrication from the essential fats like omega 3.

When considering fats, it is vital to appreciate the difference between those that can contribute to poor health and weight gain and those that are necessary for good health. There are a number of different types of fats including saturated, unsaturated and trans fats. Here's a quick guide.

Saturated fats

Saturated fats are found in animal products like meat and dairy and are also found in tropical oils like palm and coconut. Coconut oil has particular health benefits – we will look at this later.

The thinking used to be that saturated fat not only made you fat but also increased your risk of heart disease. But research in 2010, which combined the results of 21 studies (347,747 people, followed for up to 23 years) stated, 'There is no significant evidence for concluding that dietary saturated fat is associated with an increased risk of coronary heart disease, stroke and cardiovascular disease'[47].

As far as weight gain goes, when researchers compared a low-fat to a low-carbohydrate diet, the latter won hands down – with participants on the low-carbohydrate diet logging significantly more weight loss at six and 12 months, significantly higher HDL (good cholesterol) and lower triglycerides (fat in the blood)[48].

In my opinion, saturated fat does not cause weight gain. But it is found in many foods that are not good for your health – fatty and processed meats like sausages and bacon, as well as foods high in refined carbohydrates like pastries and cakes. I'm convinced by the evidence that saturated fat alone doesn't increase cholesterol or heart disease risk. But I concur with the NHS recommendation that women should eat no more than 20g of saturated fat a day and men no more 30g a day[49].

People always ask me whether they should use butter or margarine/low-fat spreads. Personally, I choose organic butter as I think it is a more natural product. Butter is made by churning cream and if you buy an unsalted version there is only one ingredient on the label – butter. A typical margarine, though, could have a list of ingredients including sunflower oil, palm oil, water, salt, emulsifiers, flavour, regulator of acidity, colour, vitamin A, vitamin D. For me this is a refined, processed food because sunflower oil is liquid at room temperature so something has to be done to the oil to make it solid. It's also an omega 6 fat and I believe most of us have too many of these in our diets (compared to the omega 3 fats we need more of, see page 65). Hard margarines can also contain trans fats.

Coconut oil

This deserves a special mention because the nutrition world has changed its view on coconut oil in recent years. Yes, it does contain a high amount of saturated fat (over 90 per cent, which is more than butter), but two thirds of this fat comes in the form of medium chain fatty acids (also known as medium chain triglycerides or MCT), mainly lauric acid. Dairy products for instance only contain about ten to 12 per cent MCTs. Lauric acid can be easily converted into energy by the body, instead of being stored as fat. It's also been suggested that coconut oil could help with weight loss because it is promotes thermogenesis, increasing metabolism and producing energy.

Coconut oil, like other saturated fats, can safely be used for cooking even at high temperatures. It can't be damaged in the same way as polyunsaturated oils which can create free radicals (linked to premature ageing, cancer and heart disease) when heated to a high temperature.

Unsaturated fats

Unsaturated fats include essential fatty acids, which are a vital component of every human cell. Your body needs them to insulate nerve cells, keep your skin and arteries supple, balance hormones and keep you warm.

Essential fatty acids are found in nuts, seeds, beans, oily fish and egg yolks.

Unsaturated fats fall into two main groups: monounsaturated and polyunsaturated.

Monounsaturated fats are so called because, chemically speaking, they only have one double bond. These are known as omega 9 fats and olive oil is high in these fats.

Polyunsaturated fats can have two or more double bonds and these are the essential fats because your body cannot produce them. Within this group there is a further split into omega 6 and omega 3 fatty acids. These oils should have an ideal balance in your body.

Omega 6 oils are found in sunflower, corn, sesame, evening primrose oil and borage oils. Omega 3s are found in oily fish, flaxseeds (linseeds), soya and walnuts. Omega 3 oils are often lacking in our diet, but they are very beneficial to your health, as they have been found to enhance immune function, improve energy levels and soften the skin. They also increase your metabolic rate, so adding omega 3 oils to your eating plan can actually help you to lose weight.

Your body makes beneficial prostaglandins (hormone-like regulating substances) from omega 3s. These are particularly useful as they help lower blood pressure, decrease inflammation and decrease sodium and water retention.

Signs of a lack of omega 3 fatty acids in your diet include dry skin, lifeless hair, cracked nails, fatigue, depression, dry eyes, lack of motivation, aching joints, difficulty in losing weight, forgetfulness and breast pain. If you have tried to lose weight by going on a low-fat or no-fat diet, you are likely to be deficient in these essential fats. It is now estimated that we obtain up to 25 times more omega 6 fats from our diet than omega 3s. Over the past century there has been an 80 per cent decrease in their consumption.

Before you consider taking any omega-oil supplements, be sure to read Chapter 7 and the section on Omega 3, 6 and 9 oils, as it's important to take the right ones.

Trans fats

Trans fats are the worst kind of fat possible. They are found in processed foods such as cakes and biscuits, deep-fried and fast foods and have no benefit to our health – rather they can harm it. Since 2008, UK manufacturers have stopped using trans fats as an ingredient in foods but any food that is manufactured outside the UK but sold in the UK can still contain them.

Trans fats are chemically altered liquid oils that have hydrogen passed through them at a high temperature and high pressure, to turn them into solids (this gives them a longer shelf life). Look out for the words 'hydrogenated' or 'partially hydrogenated vegetable oil' on a food label. If the label just says 'vegetable oil' then it won't contain trans fats.

Trans fats can increase your risk of heart disease because they increase bad cholesterol (LDL) and decrease good cholesterol (HDL). If you increase your consumption of trans fats by just 2 per cent you can increase your risk of heart disease by a massive 30 per cent[50]. These fats can also block the absorption of the essential fats.

Trans fats make your cells harden and lose their elasticity which is not good news for your arteries or your brain (which is 70 per cent fat). It is also very bad news for your insulin receptors. If your insulin receptors become resistant then it is harder to lose weight because you are producing more of the fat-storing hormone insulin and can increase your risk of developing type 2 diabetes.

What happens during the process of hydrogenation?

1. Vegetable oil is mixed thoroughly with fine particles of nickel or copper.
2. The oil is heated to approximately 200 degrees centigrade and held at that heat for six hours.
3. Meanwhile, hydrogen gas is pumped through the mixture at high pressure and the excited hydrogen atoms penetrate the vegetable oil molecules and chemically change them into 'trans fats'. These are new, complex substances that are not found in nature, except at low levels in some animal fats.
4. The mixture must be kept very hot – if it cools down at this stage the whole production line will become clogged.
5. The mixture is then cooled down to form tiny hard plastic-like beads, known as hydrogenated oil.
6. The beads of hydrogenated oil are mixed with liquid oil and heated up again to a high temperature. When this cools you have a solid fat.

Because these trans fats are not natural and have a plastic-like quality, your body has great difficulty in trying to eliminate or utilise them. So, instead, it stores them as excess fat. Your body is then put under extra pressure just to deal with a substance that you do not really need to eat.

A number of countries and US states have now banned the use of foods containing trans fats, including Denmark, Switzerland, New York, California and Austria.

Choosing and using oils

Careful choice, storage and use of oils is essential as they can easily be damaged by a process called oxidation. This leaves the oil open to attack by highly reactive chemical fragments called free radicals. Free radicals have been linked to cancer, coronary heart disease, rheumatoid arthritis and premature ageing. Free radicals speed up the ageing process by destroying healthy cells as well as attacking collagen (the 'cement' that holds our cells together), which is the primary organic constituent of bone, cartilage and connective tissue. Collagen naturally decreases with age, resulting in certain changes to your body:

- skin can become wrinkled
- veins are more prominent
- wounds may heal more slowly
- you bruise more easily
- nails may become brittle
- eyes feel dry and develop dark circles underneath
- gums may bleed or become prone to infection
- hair can look dull with split ends, grow less and maybe even fall out
- bad breath and mouth ulcers develop

Anyone over 40 has almost certainly experienced one or more of these but if we can decrease our exposure to free radicals we can reduce the incidence of such problems.

The following measures can help:

- Choose cold-pressed, unrefined vegetable oils or extra-virgin olive oil, organic where possible. Unfortunately, most supermarket oils are manufactured with chemicals and heat so that the maximum amount of oil is extracted from each batch. This destroys the quality of the oil and its nutritional content. Anti-foaming agents may also have been added to the oils.
- Do not fry polyunsaturated fats such as sunflower oil. They can become more easily oxidised when heated as they have more than one chemical bond, hence the term 'poly'. Choose butter or coconut oil instead. Butter (including ghee) and coconut oils do not create free radicals when heated to high temperatures because they are saturated.
- If cooking at lower temperatures you can also use monounsaturated olive oil which has less chance of creating free radicals because it only has one chemical bond, hence 'mono'. Reduce temperature to minimise oxidation.
- Keep all fats to a minimum when frying; try to bake or grill instead.
- Rapeseed oil (known as canola oil in the US) can be heated to higher temperatures but I personally don't use it. As a crop it seems to require many more chemicals than others to help it to grow and is very vulnerable to insects so lots of pesticides are used in its production, too. These chemicals can run off the fields into our water supply, polluting streams and rivers. A 2017 report by the Health and Safety Executive Pesticides Forum says that the main pesticides which results in our water quality standards being compromised are the herbicides used to protect rapeseed crops[51]. But the chemicals used to spray the crop are not only affecting our water

supply but can also be affecting the bee population and bees are very attracted to rapeseed because of its rich source of pollen and nectar. Until recently, a pesticide called neonicotinoid was used on the rapeseed crop and it affects the bees' ability to forage, navigate and reproduce. In 2018 the EU has now voted in favour of an almost total ban on the use of neonicotinoid insecticides outdoors. They can still be used indoors in greenhouses to treat crops. Manufacturers and certain farming groups are not happy with the ban and this has led to a decrease of rapeseed being grown in the EU, but it can be imported from outside Europe, where it can still be treated with neonicotinoids. If you are going to use rapeseed oil then absolutely make sure it is organic.

- Do not store oils in clear bottles on a window sill as light can cause free radical damage. Choose oils in dark glass bottles (or decant into them) and keep them shut away in a cupboard.

Supplementing omega 3 essential fats

If you find it difficult to eat oily fish or you are a vegan or vegetarian then you might need to supplement with omega 3s, in order to make sure you are getting enough.

I will explain in more detail in Chapter 7, but the important part of the omega 3s are the EPA (eicosapentaenoic acid) and (DHA) docosahexaenoic acid which are naturally found in oily fish. Research shows most of the crucial health benefits come from EPA and DHA.

It is possible to get your omega 3s from a plant source like flaxseeds, either in food form or in a supplement like flaxseed oil. But it is in the form of ALA (alpha-linolenic acid), which your body has to convert to EPA and DHA. There's more on supplementing if you're vegan in Chapter 7.

7. Increase your natural fibre intake

Fibre in its natural form is helpful in balancing blood sugar levels, but it is mainly known for its action on the bowel and the beneficial effect it has on problems like constipation.

- Soluble fibre is found in oats, nuts, seeds, beans and some fruits and vegetables. It attracts water and slows down your digestion.
- Insoluble fibre is found in whole grains. It makes the stool more bulky to help food pass more efficiently through the digestive tract.

Fibre binds to water and increases the bulk of your stools, so that they are easier to eliminate from your body. It also prevents putrefaction of food which can result if food stays in your bowel too long. Putrefying food will ferment, causing a build-up of gas, leading to problems like bloating and flatulence.

Fibre also increases your feeling of fullness and removes toxins from your body. By filling you up it helps you to feel more satisfied with what you have eaten and lessens the tendency to overeat. Other health benefits include a reduction in diseases of the bowel (including bowel cancer) and reduced cholesterol levels.

Fibre also determines how much oestrogen is stored and how much is excreted – soluble fibre binds to oestrogen so that it is excreted efficiently. As such, chronic constipation has been linked to breast cancer as it has been shown that regular bowel motions are associated with more excretion of oestrogen and lower levels in the blood[52]. Toxic waste products that are not eliminated properly can end up stored in your body's fatty tissue, including the breasts.

Fibre also increases the amount of time you spend chewing food, hence slowing down eating. The first part of digestion starts in your mouth so chew well and your food will be digested better. (Also, your brain takes 20 minutes to register that you are full so by eating more slowly you will consume less food and still be satisfied, which is a great way to automatically reduce your portion size.)

Beware of bran as a source of fibre

Two English doctors, Denis Burkitt and Hugh Trowell, alerted the world to the health benefits of high-fibre foods in the 1960s. They had spent many years working in Africa where they noticed that Africans had a much lower level of diseases such as bowel cancer than Europeans. They linked this to the Africans' very high-fibre diet and made a connection between plenty of fibre and better health. The Africans' source of fibre came from whole grains (not wheat) and fruit. Unfortunately, many people misinterpreted the theory and believed we should add bran to food to increase the fibre content – wheat bran was seen as a convenient source of fibre in the UK because it was readily available and relatively cheap, as it is a by-product of grain milling.

Bran, however, counts as a refined food because it is contained in the grains of cereal plants and then striped away to be sold on its own. It contains phytates which have a binding effect on certain vital nutrients such as iron, zinc, calcium and magnesium, making it less easy for the body to absorb them. Eating bran has led to gastrointestinal problems such as bloating and flatulence. It makes much more sense to eat the bran in the form that nature intended by eating the grains in their whole state.

Recommendations for increasing natural fibre in your diet

Include:

- Plenty of fresh fruit and vegetables (cooked and raw).
- Whole grains like brown rice, wholegrain bread and crackers, oats, barley, millet, spelt, buckwheat, amaranth.
- Pulses in salads or in cooking (tinned for convenience are fine but do check the label for hidden sugar). Always soak dried pulses and rinse and drain both dried and tinned.
- Nuts and seeds.
- Muesli – soak it first for at least 10 minutes (overnight is best) as it contains raw flakes of various grains. Soaking enables the phytates to be broken down so they do not affect mineral absorption. If you are buying a ready-made muesli, always check the label for added sugars as some can be deceptively and unnecessarily sweet. Dried fruit is OK but you don't want any refined sugar added.

Avoid or reduce:

- Refined carbohydrates including cakes, bread and biscuits and everything containing white flour and sugar.
- Bran on its own or in breakfast cereals.

Constipation

If you are not going to the toilet every day and/or your stools are hard to pass then you are constipated. It is important that your bowels are working properly because their function is to get rid of everything that your body doesn't need. If you are not eliminating toxins and poisons efficiently they can be reabsorbed into your system and cause ill health.

Start by increasing your intake of fresh fruit and vegetables: this should make quite a difference fairly quickly. And make sure you are drinking good amounts of water each day (6-8 glasses, herbal teas will count). If you still need more help to go to the toilet comfortably and regularly, then soak a tablespoon (15ml) of whole flaxseeds in a small amount of water for around 30 minutes and then swallow with the water used for soaking and some extra water just before you go to bed.

The soaked flaxseeds form a mucilaginous substance which is moist and sticky and helps your stools to slip easily and smoothly through the bowel and out the other end. The action of the flaxseeds is very mild so can even be used in the long term.

Vitamin C can also be used to help soften stools. Try adding a supplement of 500mg twice a day and increase by 500mg at a time until your stools are manageable, soft and comfortable (a good alkaline form of vitamin C I use in the clinic is NHP's Vitamin C Support (see www.naturalhealthpractice.com).

8. Reduce salt in your diet

Salt (sodium chloride) is the major source of sodium in your body. Sodium is a mineral that is closely connected with your body's ability to balance water retention and blood pressure. The higher the level of blood sodium, the higher the blood pressure. Another mineral, potassium, works with sodium to regulate your water balance and normalise your heart rhythm. The more sodium you consume, the more potassium you need to counteract this effect. So you need to do two things: reduce your loss of potassium and reduce your intake of sodium.

Potassium loss can be caused by diuretics and laxatives. Low blood sugar can also cause potassium loss as it stimulates the uptake of potassium from the blood stream[53].

Alcohol, coffee and sugar also make us lose potassium so here's another good reason to reduce these stimulants.

Sodium reduction can be effectively achieved by reducing your intake of salt. Salt is added to most of our ready-prepared foods, including tomato ketchup, salad dressings, biscuits, pizzas. It is better to get out of the habit of adding salt to food at the table, as it is often added during cooking and more is not needed.

The World Health Organisation wants us to achieve an intake of less than 5g of salt (1 teaspoon of salt, approximately 2g of sodium) per day by the year 2025. At the moment the target is 6g (1 rounded teaspoon salt, 2.4g of sodium) and if we could achieve this it would save 17,000 lives a year because of the reduction in blood pressure, preventing strokes, heart attacks and heart failure.

We only need 0.5g of sodium a day to keep us healthy. Some people can end up eating 9g of salt a day and it is easy to consume too much without realising. One burger in a bun can contain 6g, two slices of wholemeal bread 1.2g and a slice of cheese and tomato pizza 5.3g. Two slices of bread can contain more salt than a packet of crisps. Always read food labels carefully to check for the presence of salt.

We also consume sodium as sodium nitrate which is the preservatives used in meat and as monosodium glutamate, the flavour enhancer, often used in convenience and Chinese foods. Food which is advertised as low fat or low sugar can be extremely high in salt to give it flavour.

There are now quite a number of different salts to choose from, e.g. table salt, rock salt, sea salt, Himalayan salt, low salt. First of all I would suggest avoiding regular table salt as these will often contain anti-caking agents to stop the salt clumping together so that it flows more easily. In the UK, sodium ferrocyanide and potassium ferrocyanide are often used in table salt as the anti-caking agents.

Sea salt is made by evaporating sea water and in theory should contain some trace nutrients like zinc. Himalayan salt is pink in colour (coming from the iron content) and is mined from a salt mine in Pakistan.

One study analysed the minerals levels of 38 different types of salt. The sodium levels of the different salts were pretty much equal and the Himalayan salt had higher levels of potassium than the other salts. Some of the sea salts had higher levels of magnesium and calcium than the Himalayan but the differences were very small. The lowest levels of minerals other than sodium were found in the table salt[54].

Best to avoid table salt but the artisan salts are very similar in sodium content. There are some potassium salts which contain both sodium and potassium chloride and have 70 per cent less sodium than table salt. This type of salt may be helpful for someone with high blood pressure but if you have kidney disease or diabetes then you would need to check with doctor as it may not be good to increase your potassium intake.

Recommendations to reduce sodium intake:

- Choose more freshly prepared foods so that you are aware of all the ingredients.
- Use herbs, garlic, ginger, cinnamon, turmeric, lemon juice and other spices in cooking to add flavour.
- Read labels carefully for hidden salt.
- Avoid or cut right down on salt added at the table or in cooking.
- Avoid convenience or prepared foods with a high salt content – the food should not contain 0.5g of more of sodium (1.25g salt) per 100g.

• Chapter 4 •

Shop and Cook Wisely

The key to shopping is simple: buy your food in its most natural state. Ask yourself what had happened to the food or drink before it reached the shops. Try to buy organic produce that has not been sprayed with pesticides and herbicides as these can act as endocrine-disrupting chemicals and upset the delicate male and female hormone balance.

Ideally, your food should come without ingredient labels – as whole foods. But I accept that few of us have time to create all our food from scratch. So you need to become a label detective.

If ever there were labels that mattered it's the ones on the food we eat. Yet most of us lead busy lives with little time to spare for reading the small print on food labels. It's definitely a habit worth getting into though. Once you begin reading labels you could be in for a big surprise – you probably had no idea you were putting so many chemicals into your body. OK, your supermarket shop may take longer the first couple of times. You'll have to get used to the ingredient terms used and brand differences. You may even find it useful to make notes that you can refer to as you shop. But, once you are familiar with the best brands to buy, whizzing round the aisles for the healthiest foods will become a breeze.

How to check a food label

The ingredients on a label are listed with the first ingredient having the greatest quantity and the last having the least quantity in that product. Unfortunately, most labels do not tell us exactly how much of each ingredient is in the food: so one fish pie could contain more fish than another and we wouldn't know.

It is best to avoid ingredients which sound like a chemistry lesson. For example, these are the contents of one brand of apricot dessert:

sugar, hydrogenated vegetable oil, gelling agents (E331, E401, E431), emulsifiers (E447, E322), adipic acid, lactose, caseinate, whey powder, flavourings, artificial sweetener, colours (E110, E122, E102, E160a).

So we immediately know that the ingredient with the greatest quantity in this dessert is sugar. But have you spotted something even more important? Where are the apricots? Common sense should tell us that this isn't a very natural or healthy food.

E-numbers

As a general guide, I recommend you avoid products with E-numbers. Some are fine to eat, as they are naturally derived, but the vast majority are not and many have known side effects. There are books on the market that provide E-number references and websites that list them. If you are very diligent, you could check them when shopping – but that could become tedious and time-consuming. The best action is simply to avoid the processed products containing them.

E-numbers include permitted colours (some natural, some not), preservatives, permitted antioxidants (some natural, such as ascorbic acid or vitamin C, others not), emulsifiers and stabilisers, sweeteners, solvents, mineral hydrocarbons and modified starches. Some products might list natural annatto colouring on the label, for instance. This is labelled E160b and has no known adverse side effects.

Artificial sweeteners

Let's be very clear here. Artificial sweeteners are chemicals and the safety of many of them is in doubt. They are best avoided. Artificial sweeteners are used in a wide variety of foods and drinks. They have an obvious advantage for manufacturers in that they are much cheaper than sugar and, in some, cases, sweeter. Saccharin, for instance, is 300 times sweeter than sugar.

As I've already warned, the danger of these sweeteners lies not only in their individual effects but also the chemical cocktail that may result from consuming a number of varying sweeteners in different foods and drinks over a day. The artificial sweeteners you are likely to encounter in no-sugar, low-sugar or diet foods or drinks include saccharin, aspartame, acesulfame K and sucralose.

Most people use artificial sweeteners when wanting to lose weight because they contain no calories. I accept this is tempting. However, I really want you to realise that they are not a good solution. Not only are they far from natural, and may have serious health concerns attached, but as far as weight loss goes, they may actually help *prevent* it. Sweeteners can change your appetite.

We touched on this earlier in the book but let's recap. Normally when you eat something sweet, your body expects a bulk of calories to come with that food. However, artificial sweeteners are sweet with no calories so you actually get an increase in appetite in order to prompt you to obtain those calories from somewhere else. So artificial sweeteners can make you gain weight, because you end up eating more and it doesn't eliminate your sweet tooth.

Sugar activates the sweet receptors on your tongue and increases dopamine in your brain and the artificial sweeteners also have this effect. But sugar has a secondary effect when it causes an increase in glucose. Artificial sweeteners have no effect on your blood sugar or may even give you low blood sugar (hypoglycaemia), which leaves you feeling hungry, unsatisfied with what you have eaten, making you eat more the next time.

When rats are fed artificial sweeteners they take in more calories, weigh more and, even more worryingly, this weight is made up of an increase in body fat percentage[55].

Two groups of rats were given exactly the same amount of calories, but one group was given either saccharin or aspartame (artificial sweeteners) and the other group was given sugar (sucrose). The rats given the artificial sweeteners gained more weight than rats eating sugar[56]. So even if you think you can control your appetite and you are not eating more when using artificial sweeteners you are still going to gain weight.

And it is not only your weight that can be affected. Research on more than 400,000 people over 10 years showed that not only did they gain weight, but they had an increased risk of type 2 diabetes and heart disease[57].

Artificial sweeteners can have a negative effect on the beneficial bacteria in your gut[58]. We already know that gut bacteria have a role to play in insulin resistance, obesity, non-alcohol fatty liver disease and type 2 diabetes[59] and that there is a difference in the gut bacteria composition in normal and overweight people[60].

Be very wary of labels which say 'no added sugar', 'low sugar', 'light/lite' or 'diet' – usually these mean that an artificial sweetener has been added instead of sugar.

Sugar may also be broken down into a number of sugars in the ingredient list. This is a manufacturer's trick to avoid grouping them together and having to list sugar as the first (and therefore greatest) ingredient. Sugar can be broken down into: sucrose, fructose, glucose, dextrose, maltodextrin, lactose, maltose and corn syrup. In one breakfast cereal there may be five different sugars listed in the ingredients.

Small is beautiful

Generally, the longer the ingredients list, the more suspicious you should be about the origin of the product. Manufacturers argue that additives, preservatives and flavourings, and so on, are used in such small quantities that they will not have any adverse effect. However, when you take into account all the small amounts in all the different products we eat and drink every day, these small amounts soon add up. I believe we're unwittingly creating a chemical cocktail inside ourselves – and nobody knows exactly how these chemicals will react together.

It is quite impossible to make sure every morsel you eat is chemical free, especially if your lifestyle means you have to take snacks or meals away from home, as most of us do. Just make sure that what you eat at home is as natural and healthy as possible. 'Everything in moderation' is the best rule to follow. If your busy life means that sometimes you have to buy convenience or packaged food, then find the best brand you can and go for the shortest, least chemical-looking ingredients list possible.

Tips for preparation and cooking

- Organic root vegetables and tubers such as carrots, sweet potatoes, parsnips, swede and potatoes only need scrubbing. Do not peel them as many of the nutrients are concentrated just under the skin.

- Lightly cook vegetables in a little water or steam.

- Avoid high temperature frying and especially deep frying where possible because of the possibility of free radical damage to the oil (see previous chapter). Try baking or steam frying. To steam fry, use a little oil to sauté your vegetables in a wok or frying pan, and then add a little water or stock to the pan and cover it with a lid. The steam from the liquid cooks the food, you can then take off the lid when the food is cooked and let the rest of the liquid boil off.

- Choose your cookware with care. Avoid aluminium, as this is a toxic heavy metal that can enter the food though the cooking[61]. Avoid any coated cookware, such as non-stick, as animal studies show it could be carcinogenic[62]. Perfluorooctanoic acid (PFOA) is widely used in the manufacture of non-stick coatings and research shows that PFOA has been detected in the blood of more than 98 per cent of the US population[63]. Researchers aren't sure if this enters via chemicals used in non-stick pans and/or via environmental pollution. The best move is to stop using non-stick cookware altogether or to reduce the risk of the non-stick coating eroding or flaking into your food use only a low or medium heat and avoid using abrasive cleaners, metal scourers or metal utensils. Overheated non-stick pans can also emit poisonous fumes so never leave dry or empty non-stick pans on hot burners. The best cookware materials are cast iron, enamel, glass, copper and stainless steel.

- Be careful of microwaving. I do have concerns about microwaving as a cooking method. My understanding is that it does not destroy the water soluble vitamins, like C and the B vitamins but destroys the fat soluble ones (A, D and E). A microwave heats food by using high-frequency electromagnetic waves, similar to TV. The molecules of the food agitate at over 2,000 times per second so that the food heats itself.

In traditional methods of cooking, infrared waves heat the food and the heat is transferred from the pot to the food or directly from the heat as in grilling. The food is cooked in a slower, gentler way than in microwaving. It is thought that the process of microwaving can create more free radical damage in the food. Free radicals are highly reactive chemicals which are linked to cancer, coronary heart disease and premature ageing.

My other concern with microwaving is the reaction with plastic containers. Many plastic containers contain endocrine disrupting chemicals (EDCs) such as Bisphenol A (BPA), which can disrupt hormones by interfering with the production or utilisation of a person's own hormones or by mimicking the action of the hormones.

The problem is that these EDCs are more likely to be transferred from the plastic to the food when the plastic is heated and also if the food contains fat as these EDCs are lipophilic (fat-loving) and will migrate more easily into fat.

Shopping list

Variety is the key to enjoying your food and eating for health and weight control. There may be foods mentioned below that you have never tried – if so, experiment and enjoy yourself. In an ideal world, we would all shop at small retailers offering local, organic produce but that isn't always practical. If you can support your local shops, wholefood store, organic farm shop or farmers' market or independent health food store, then do – your food will contain far less food miles and your support will be far more helpful to the local economy. However many of us will have to rely on supermarkets or home deliveries.

The following is your shopping list for foods that will help you keep your weight under control.

Fruit

Fresh fruit, organic where possible, is a great health staple. Many supermarkets sell seasonal organic fruit and you may even find frozen organic fruit. It can be slightly more expensive but in health terms is well worth the extra cost. It also tastes better. If you live in a rural area hunt down a local organic farm shop or look out for organic delivery firms. It can be a challenge to get all your fruit organic but just do what you can. Sometimes it may just be organic apples that you can get and the rest will be non-organic. If price or availability is a factor, better to go organic if you eat the whole fruit (apples, berries), and non-organic if you peel them (oranges and bananas). If you have the time you could consider growing some fruits yourself – apart from the fact that they make your garden look delightful you also know for sure that your produce is pesticide-free.

Make sure you eat a wide variety of fruit, don't just choose your old favourites week in, week out. Eat seasonally and look for what's grown locally. But also take advantage of the fact we have a myriad of tropical treats on offer these days – look for something new that you haven't tasted before every time you shop.

Just be careful of fruits with a high GI while you are getting your weight under control (these include bananas, pineapple and melon). If you do eat high GI fruits then take them in moderation and remember to include a protein with them (for example, nuts or seeds) which will lower the GI of the fruit.

Fruit is very versatile. It can be enjoyed raw or mashed up into natural live yogurt and is ideal any time of the day. If you need to snack away from home it's easy to carry and is good for children's lunch boxes. You can always use frozen fruit if you don't have fresh fruit to hand or its out of season (or cheaper!). Tinned fruit is better than not having any fruit, but always buy it tinned in natural juice or water, not syrup.

Dried fruit

Raisins, apricots, dates, sultanas, prunes, figs, apple rings, mango strips, pineapple crisps – the list of dried fruit we can buy these days is getting longer and more exotic. Dried fruits make an enjoyable change but eat them in moderation as the drying process makes the sugar more concentrated. Once again, it's better to eat them with protein. So if you are craving chocolate mid-afternoon try having some nuts and raisins instead. The raisins will satisfy the sweet craving and the nuts will lower the GI of the raisins. With the raisins and other dried fruit keep to one heaped tablespoon per day.

When buying dried fruit, avoid any that contain the preserving agent sulphur dioxide which is also used as a bleaching agent in flour. Sulphur dioxide occurs naturally but is produced chemically for commercial use. It's used most often on dried apricots to keep them a 'nice' orange colour (figs and dates tend to be sulphur dioxide-free). The packet will state whether or not they are free from sulphur dioxide. Those that are free from this preservative will look brown rather than bright apricot but taste fine.

Supermarket dried fruits such as mixed fruit, raisins and sultanas will often have mineral oil added to them. This gives them a shiny appearance and keeps them separate. Try to avoid these as the oil can interfere with the absorption of calcium and phosphorus. As it passes through your body, mineral oil can pick up and excrete the oil-soluble vitamins (A, D, E, K), which you really want to retain. You will need to check the ingredient list to see whether mineral oil had been added.

Vegetables and salads

Everybody knows about the five-a-day fruit and vegetable target but you should actually aim to eat more vegetables than fruit. Vegetables give you the most benefits for your health but it is often easier just to pick up a piece of fruit. Apparently, the UK five-a-day target came about because the Government thought that was something most people might manage but research has shown that only one in four adults are actually eating five a day. Interestingly, in other countries the targets are different. In Denmark it is six a day. Canada suggests five to 10 while the US advises eight to 10. In Australia and Japan they break down the amount of vegetables and fruit with the emphasis on more vegetables. So for Australia the target is five portions of vegetables and two of fruit; in Japan it's a whopping 13 vegetables and four portions of fruit.

Research from Imperial College London suggests that our five-a-day target should be increased to 10. This could reduce the chance of having a stroke by a third, the risk of heart disease by 24 per cent and the risk of dying prematurely by 31 per cent. Not all fruit and vegetables carried the same benefits, according to the study. Apples, pears, citrus fruit, salads and green leafy vegetables such as lettuce and chicory, and cruciferous vegetables such as broccoli, cabbage and cauliflower were found to be the best at preventing heart disease and stroke. There did not seem to be any difference in the protective effects of cooked versus raw fruit and vegetables[64].

So my message is to increase your intake of vegetables and, as with fruit, enjoy as wide a variety of as possible. Go for a rainbow of colours and you'll increase the range of nutrients you're taking in (many of the vitamins and antioxidants are contained in the pigments). Pick a new veg to try each week. Remember that potatoes do not count as one of your five-a-day due to a high starch content.

Grains

If your budget limits the amount of organic produce you can buy, put grains at the top of the shopping list. Grains are very small so will absorb more pesticides than other goods, so it is best to buy organic. You will have no trouble buying organic grains at health food shops although many supermarkets now stock them, too.

Include barley, bulgur, brown basmati rice, buckwheat (not technically a grain), couscous, millet, oats, brown rice, quinoa (cooks like a grain but is a high-protein seed), spelt and other ancient grains like kamut and amaranth.

Go for variety with grains as much as you do with veg and fruit. Experiment with new varieties, don't just stick to pasta and rice. If you feel bloated after eating wheat, then limit your intake even of whole wheat and the same would apply to bulgur and couscous. Spelt is a strain of wheat but is often called 'ancient wheat' because it is one of the original strains of wheat. Spelt is much easier to digest than wheat so you might find that you get on better with it in this form.

If you are a home baker you will find there are a wide range of wholegrain flours to choose from for bread and pastry baking, some are even gluten-free.

There are a number of wholegrain pastas available and you can also buy buckwheat and rice noodles and pastas made from quinoa, spelt, corn and vegetables.

Bread

As always, organic is best and choose wholegrain where possible. Read the labels as even some wholemeal bread can contain sugar and flour improvers.

You can also buy rye bread, some will contain wheat and others contain 100 per cent rye. There is also a growing amount of bread being baked with more unusual combinations of grains. Spelt bread is now particularly popular and also sourdough and seeded breads.

Crackers

If you want something lighter than bread, then there is a wide variety of wholegrain crackers available at supermarkets and health food shops. You can also buy organic ones. Wholewheat, spelt, rye, oats, rice and buckwheat crackers are available.

Flavourings

Choose from ginger, garlic, fresh and dried herbs, spices like cinnamon, turmeric, pepper and chilli, lemon juice, sea salt, miso (soya bean paste), mustard (check for added sugar, artificial additives).

Arrowroot or kuzu are good for thickening gravies and sauces.

You can find tomato ketchup without sugar and also no-added-sugar mayonnaise and salad dressings. Or make your own.

Soy or soya sauce. Not just for Chinese food, this is good on rice, in vegetable stir-fries and in salad dressings and sauces. Choose organic where possible and avoid those containing monosodium glutamate. If you are avoiding wheat then buy tamari, which is a wheat- and gluten-free soya sauce.

Nuts

You can enjoy almonds, Brazil nuts, cashews, hazelnuts, pecans, pine kernels, pistachios and walnuts. Try to have the nuts in their raw form, and not roasted or coated in honey or salt. You can also buy nut milks like almond and hazelnut milk. There are also some delicious nut butters, not just peanut butter – try almond, cashew nut, brazil nut – that you can use as spreads. You will need to read the ingredients as some nut butters add sugar or palm oil. You just want the nuts blended up.

Nuts can be eaten as a snack or used in cooking or salads. Pine nuts added to brown rice during cooking make a healthy and enjoyable change.

Seeds

Try chia, sunflower, sesame, pumpkin, poppy and caraway. They can be added to salads or cooked vegetable dishes or put in with rice when cooking. You can have a combination of nuts and seeds as a snack. They can be added to muesli, ground and sprinkled on porridge and you can also get seed butters now such as pumpkin seed butter to use as a spread. Try tahini (creamed sesame seeds) as a spread, in salad dressings and for making hummus.

Sweeteners

It is better to rely on the natural sweetness of foods themselves than to use sugar or artificial sweeteners. You are aiming to retrain your taste buds so that you do not need foods with added refined sugar. But if you find yourself pulled towards something sweet then it is better to go for a natural ingredient that provides sweetness alongside other nutrients.

If you are making cakes, try adding carrots, raisins or bananas to sweeten them. For apple pies or crumbles, use eating apples instead of cooking apples so that you do not need to add sugar – you could always add raisins or sultanas to make a pie or crumble sweeter. Date slice is wonderful because dates are naturally sweet. As your taste buds grow accustomed to doing without the very powerful taste of refined sugar you will come to appreciate the natural sweetness of vegetables and fruits.

There is so much confusion around 'natural' sweeteners that I am going to cover the choices in more detail.

Honey

Although this is a natural sweetener, you should only use this sparingly. Honey gets absorbed into your blood stream quickly so it is not good if you are trying to lose weight. If you are using honey then avoid types which are 'blended' or the 'produce of more than one country' because they are often heated to temperatures as high as 71 degrees C (160 degrees F) which destroys their natural goodness.

Maple syrup

Maple syrup is made from drilling a hole in the maple tree and collecting the sweet sap that drips out.

Research presented at the American Chemical Society's National Meeting in California in 2011 has suggested that maple syrup contains 34 beneficial compounds which have antioxidant and anti-inflammatory properties. A number of the syrup's antioxidant polyphenols inhibit the enzyme that converts carbohydrates to sugar, which is relevant to type 2 diabetes and weight gain. The research also showed that many of the antioxidants found in maple syrup which can help prevent the ageing of our body's cells aren't found in other natural sweeteners[65].

Maple syrup is the natural sweetener usually recommended for IBS sufferers as it causes the least problems with digestion and fermentation.

It contains significant amount of zinc and manganese and contains 15 times more calcium compared to honey.

Beware maple syrup labelled as 'maple-flavoured syrup' rather than pure 'maple syrup' as this won't be pure maple syrup and may not even contain any maple syrup at all. Ingredients of one of these maple flavoured syrups includes invert sugar syrup, colour (150d) and maple flavouring while another one has water (as its first, main, ingredient), caramel colour, alcohol, vanilla extract (vanilla bean extractives in water, alcohol and corn syrup), molasses solids, corn syrup solids, natural and artificial flavour, sugar and sulphating agents. That is why it is so important to read labels - you have to know what you are putting into your body.

Real maple syrup will be more expensive but you will only be using small amounts.

Barley malt syrup

This is an unrefined natural sweetener produced from sprouted barley. It is thick and dark brown and makes wonderful flapjacks. It is a reasonably good source of some minerals and vitamins.

Brown rice syrup

This syrup is available in most health food shops and is made from cooked brown rice cultured with enzymes to turn the starches in the rice into sugar. It contains small amounts of calcium and potassium.

Agave

This sweetener has become very popular over the last few years. In theory it should be a good natural sweetener as it comes from the agave plant in Mexico where the sap would have been boiled for hours to get the sweet syrup. The trouble is that when something becomes commercially produced on a large scale often corners are cut to make a product financially viable. It seems that to produce agave on a commercial scale the agave is made from the root bulb and the final product is just refined fructose (see below). It is even said that the fructose content is higher than the high fructose corn syrup which has had such a bad press in the US.

There will some companies who produce the agave syrup in a more traditional way but it is not easy to tell given the marketing hype around the products. I would avoid it unless it is clear that it is made traditionally.

Fructose

You can buy fructose as a white powder just like sucrose (table sugar) to add to food as a sweetener. People tend to think that fructose is fine as it is the fruit sugar naturally found in fruit. The problem is that when it is sold as a white powder it has been totally refined and all the goodness and fibre that would be in the fruit is absent.

Interestingly, fructose does not cause the release of insulin like sucrose or glucose does so it was initially thought to be a healthy form of sugar. But it has other negative effects on your health and is, therefore, best avoided.

Fructose goes straight to your liver which then has to deal with it, in the same way as alcohol. So it can make you gain weight, increase your appetite and also give you fat around the middle. Fructose gets converted into unhealthy fats such as LDL ('bad') cholesterol and triglycerides. High levels of triglycerides (blood fats) are associated with heart disease, diabetes and fatty liver disease.

Be careful also of high fructose corn syrup (HFCS), it is widely used in the US, where regular sugar costs more than in other parts of the world and HFCS is 30 per cent cheaper. It is converted from corn and can contain up to 90 per cent fructose. In the UK you can find it labelled as glucose-fructose or fructose-glucose syrup on ingredient lists and you should avoid products containing it as your liver has to do all the hard work to metabolise it.

Again you need to read labels carefully, because fructose can be used as a sweetener in many foods instead of or as well as sugar. It can also be found in food supplements especially if they are powders, in order to make the powder sweeter.

Fruit juice concentrates

These concentrates can include apple, pear, cherry and grape. Water is removed from the juice to make it concentrated and then you could just add water if you wanted to make it into a drink. In the concentrated form it can be used as a sweetener but in moderation as it is very concentrated fruit juice. The best place to use them is as a sweetener for cooking.

Stevia

Stevia is derived from the leaves of a South American plant of the same name. It is 200 to 300 times sweeter than table sugar (sucrose). Read labels carefully as many products on the market contain dextrose and flavourings – only choose 100 per cent stevia.

Stevia is not absorbed through the digestive tract so it is considered to have no calories – a good property for weight loss, you'd imagine. But although it carries no calories and is more natural than artificial sweeteners, it has the same effect of priming your body to worry about where the missing calories it associates with sweetness are. Remember what happens when that occurs? Yes. Your body will send you off to get the calories from somewhere else, increasing your appetite and causing weight gain. So I think stevia is one to avoid.

Molasses

Molasses are the byproduct of the process used to extract sugar from sugar cane or beet. Sugar cane juice is boiled and sugar crystallised. The syrup that is left over becomes molasses. Normally, the sugar cane is boiled three times to remove as much sugar as possible and the molasses left over at the end of this third stage are called black strap molasses and are dark in colour, very syrupy and have the lowest amount of sugar but the highest quantities of vitamins and minerals. But, as this is the byproduct of sugar extraction, it could contain higher levels of pesticides and other chemicals used in sugar processing. Another one to avoid unless you can find organic molasses.

Xylitol

This is another sweetener that has gained in popularity over the past few years. It is sold as a white powder and is considered natural because it occurs naturally in plants including sugar cane, corn cobs and birch. But in order to convert it into that white powder a lot of processing and refining has to take place. It is low in calories and does not need insulin to be metabolised so can be useful if you have diabetes. It also has benefits for dental health as it reduces caries. It main side effect is diarrhoea and bloating as it is a sugar alcohol and so ferments in the digestive system. I would recommend using some of the other sweeteners listed above that are less refined – unless you have diabetes and want an alternative to sugar.

Beans/legumes

With the help of good cookery books and advice from healthfood shops, you will soon find that beans, pulses and legumes are easy to cook with and very versatile. As with anything new, it is just a case of getting used to using them.

Try experimenting with aduki beans, black-eyed peas, chickpeas (used in hummus and falafel), haricot beans (used in baked beans), kidney beans, lentils (brown and red – wonderful for soups, vegetarian shepherd's pie and vegetarian spaghetti bolognese), lima beans, mung bean, navy beans, soya beans (also used for making tofu, soya sauce and miso), split peas.

Most dried beans (not lentils) need to be soaked, some overnight, before cooking. The soaking helps to remove some of the indigestible sugars that cause flatulence. Red kidney beans, especially, need to be both soaked and cooked at a high temperature for long enough (boiled for 10 minutes and then simmered for 45 minutes) otherwise they can cause food poisoning. Raw or undercooked kidney beans contain high levels of a toxin called phytohaemagglutin which is reduced to a non-toxic level by cooking.

Alternatively, you can buy beans in tins, already cooked, but watch labels for added sugar and salt and buy organic where possible. Beans make a good base for many healthy dishes, especially if you are trying to cut out meat from your eating plan – they are great added to salads, soups, stews and casseroles. Beans contain good amounts of protein, fibre and nutrients.

Many beans can also be sprouted and added to salads and stir-fries.

Fish

All fish is inherently good for you. Its saturated fat levels are low and it is very nutritious. Oily fish is particularly good as it contains high levels of omega 3 fatty acids so enjoy mackerel, fresh salmon (organic or wild, not farmed), tinned salmon (eat the bones), sardines. Avoid fish which could be high in mercury such as swordfish, marlin and fresh tuna. Tinned tuna is often produced from young tuna so does not usually contain high levels of mercury but loses the omega 3 fatty acids in the canning process. Sardines and other tinned oily fish retain their omega 3 fats even when tinned.

Eggs

Buy organic eggs where possible – free range alone isn't enough.

To be classed as free range, the hens must have had unlimited daytime access to fenced areas with vegetation and at least four square metres of outside space per bird. At night, the hens are housed in barns with bedding and perches. But there is no limit on the size of the flock. The farmers routinely trim the hen's beaks and antibiotics are regularly used.

Organically reared hens, however, cannot have their beaks trimmed, or be given hormones to make them grow quicker or routinely be given antibiotics. They have to be fed a genetically modified free diet. As the Soil Association says: 'Over 1 million tonnes of GM crops are used in the UK to feed animals which includes some free-range chickens'. Flock size is small as each organic hen has a minimum of 10 square metres of outside space.

Avoid eggs from caged or barn-reared hens for ethical as well as health reasons. Experiment too with other types of organic eggs: duck, goose, quail.

Tofu

Tofu is soya bean curd, make from yellow soya beans. On its own it has no taste: its flavour is dependent on what you cook with it. It is very versatile because of this ability to pick up the taste of whatever you combine it with and because it can be prepared in a variety of ways. It can be sliced, cubed, mashed, scrambled, pureed and used in both savoury and sweet dishes. So you can find tofu in soups, stir fries, baked in casseroles, in dips, dressings, sauces and desserts.

Add tofu to an ordinary stir fry simply by cutting it into cubes and cooking it with the other ingredients. Add strong flavours such as garlic, ginger, tamari, etc., which the tofu will absorb.

My family prefer a very simple way of eating tofu. I cut it into thin slices rather cubes and lightly fry it in olive oil. At the end of cooking, when it is pale brown and the pan is still hot, I sprinkle the tofu with tamari and gently turn it over. It is eaten as it is, often simply with brown rice and vegetables, or used in a sandwich with mayonnaise, mustard and salad.

Dairy milk alternatives

Some people find that animal milk causes them sinus problems or skin issues. It is thought that the problem is due to casein, a protein in milk, which could increase mucus production and an increase in histamine.

Even if you're fine with dairy, non-animal alternatives are generally useful to have on your shopping list. There are quite a few to choose from now including soya, almond, rice and oat milk.

With soya milk, buy organic where possible (so you know it is not genetically modified) and look for soya milk that is made from the whole beans (avoid those that mention soya isolate or soya protein isolate on the label as these are made from refined soya). When buying any of the non-dairy milks, avoid those with added sugar or preservatives.

Soya milk can be used in cooking in the same way as you would use cow's milk.

You can also easily make your own almond milk at home. It is naturally sweet and delicious in smoothies, and on cereal and porridge. Simply blend a handful of the nuts with water and strain – it will keep in the fridge for a couple of days. It's also higher in protein and nutrients than shop-bought nut milks as you'll typically use a greater proportion of nuts.

Dairy produce

As I have already said, ideally cut down your intake of dairy produce. However, if you want to continue using dairy, make sure you buy organic where possible. Buy 'live' or 'bio' yogurt. If you like fruit yogurt then add your own fruit to natural live yogurt. Frozen yogurt makes a refreshing summer dessert – use a standard recipe and substitute the sugar with maple syrup. Kefir, like yogurt, contains beneficial bacteria but it is a drink rather than a food. There are non-dairy kefir options if you prefer.

Oil/fat

See the previous chapter for more detail on oils, but to recap: organic butter is a more natural option than margarines or spread, unless you prefer a plant-based spread. Look for organic, cold-pressed, unrefined vegetable oils like sesame and sunflower. Buy organic extra virgin olive oil to use for drizzling on salads. And remember that coconut oil is safe for cooking at high temperatures (it is solid at room temperature but will swiftly melt when heated).

Tea and coffee substitutes

As a substitute for coffee try grain 'coffees' which contain various combinations of ingredients like barley, rye and chicory.

Instead of tea try herb and fruit teas, Rooibos (caffeine-free South African tea), and decaffeinated tea. Vary the herbal teas you choose to reap the benefits. Peppermint is very good for aiding digestion so it is excellent to drink after a meal. Chamomile is relaxing and is often drunk at the end of the day to help insomnia. It also has an anti-inflammatory action which is useful in the digestive system for diverticulitis as well as general colon problems.

Soft Drinks

Use real unsweetened fruit juice and dilute it 50/50 so it is not so concentrated. If a carton or bottle has 'fruit drink' on the label then you know that something else has been added. Some fruit drinks can contain only 5 per cent fruit, while the rest is made up of water, sugar and additives. You should treat flavoured spring waters with caution as many contain a surprising amount of added sugar. Liven up fruit juice with sparkling mineral water or try sparkling apple or grape juices.

Water

Let's not forget this very simple, natural drink. Our bodies are made up of approximately 70 per cent water and water is involved in every bodily process including digestion, absorption, circulation and excretion. We can survive without food for about five weeks but we can't go without water for longer than five days. Water is essential for carrying waste out of the body; it helps with constipation and also helps maintain body temperature.

Most of us do not drink nearly enough water and, ironically, if you suffer from water retention the tendency is to restrict your liquid intake thinking the less you drink, the less your body will retain. Actually, the opposite is true. If you restrict fluids, your body will try to compensate. In the same way that it will adopt a famine mode when food is restricted, it will start to retain liquid if it is concerned that fluid will be in short supply. Ideally, you should aim to drink around six glasses of water a day which should take the place of other, less healthy, drinks. Herb teas will count as a glass of water, but regular black tea and coffee don't because they have a dehydrating effect. You could start the day with a cup of hot water and a slice of lemon, a wonderfully refreshing drink and excellent for the liver.

Which water is best – tap, filtered or bottled?

Tap water is safe to drink in the UK but in some areas fluoride is added to the water supply to about 1mg of fluoride per litre of water[66]. Also research has shown certain chemicals particularly those used in dishwasher detergents are ending up in the UK drinking water (at over 10 times the level recommended by another country (Australia) for water reuse)[67].

Filtering water won't eliminate every chemical but it will help. You can buy a jug filter in which tap water is poured through a cartridge which 'cleanses' the water - but it must be changed regularly or bacteria can flourish. Alternatively, you can have a filter plumbed into your water system that will filter the water before it reaches the taps – under the kitchen sink is an ideal place. Cartridges also need changing with this system. Once you have your supply of filtered water you can use it not only for dinking but also for washing fruit and vegetables and cooking.

Bottled water comes in many guises so here is a short guide to help you understand what you are buying. Choose glass bottles (and recycle) rather than plastic – plastic can leach into the water and we all need to reduce plastic waste.

- **Spring Water** - may have been taken from one or more underground sources and have undergone a range of treatments, such as filtration and blending.
- **Natural Mineral Water** - bottled in its natural underground state and untreated in any way. It has to come from an officially registered source, conform to purity standards and carry details of its source and mineral analysis on the label.
- **Naturally Sparkling Water** – water from its underground source with enough natural carbon dioxide to make it bubbly.
- **Sparkling (Carbonated) Water** – has had carbon dioxide added to it during bottling, the same as with ordinary fizzy drinks.

Convenience foods

As discussed throughout this book, processed foods are best avoided in favour of whole foods and home cooking. But there are some exceptions that are healthy and useful to have at home when time is tight. They include baked beans, other tinned pulses (for a quick mixed-bean salad), tinned or fresh soups, miso soup powders or pastes. Just be careful to read the label for added sugar, artificial sweeteners, colourings or stabilisers like sodium phosphates, which you want to avoid. Watch out as some miso soups may contain MSG (monosodium glutamate).

Ready-prepared meals

Despite your good intentions to eat well it may sometimes be necessary to go for a ready meal. If so, look for the more wholesome types. Often frozen meals can be 'cleaner' as they don't require so many preservatives. Check for and avoid added sugar, colourings and artificial sweeteners.

Snacks

Fresh fruit, dried fruit, nuts and raisins are all good and tasty to use as a snack at any time. You can buy good quality crisps and tortilla (corn) chips from most shops. Some manufacturers use sea salt in these products. Check crisps and chips to see if the oil used is hydrogenated. If so, then buy another brand. There are good quality rye crackers and rice and oat cakes available on the market (check for added sugar).

You can buy some good quality snack bars which are just made with fruit/nuts and no added sugar so have a look in a good health food shop.

Jams

If you're partial to jam you don't need to miss out. There are some very good-quality, sugar-free jams available. (Officially the word 'jam' means a preserve, which implies that it contains sugar to act as a preservative – so the natural sugar-free jams have to be called spreads.) They contain only real fruit and a setting agent such as pectin from limes. The choice of flavours is quite amazing, including apricot, blackcurrant, kiwi, mixed berry, pineapple, plum, morello cherry, peach and passion fruit, blackberry and apple, wild blueberry, wild hedgerow and the usual strawberry and raspberry.

If you see a supermarket jam or spread marked 'sugar-free' check the label for artificial sweeteners. The jam should be made solely from fruit. There are also some excellent marmalades made purely from oranges with no added sugar.

Some jam companies have been known to extract the colour from the fruit during the jam making process and then add artificial colours to give their products a rich colour. Natural jams may not look quite as bright but they are delicious.

Because they contain no preservatives they must be kept in the fridge after opening.

Desserts

As you steer away from pre-packaged foods, it becomes more necessary to make your own desserts if, like many of us, you like something sweet to end a meal. For speed and convenience, you can eat fresh fruit either whole or cut up as a fruit salad or mixed into live yogurt. Baked eating apples are easy to prepare with a stuffing of sultanas. Stewed fruit or compotes can also be prepared easily – remember to avoid adding sugar. You'll be amazed at how quickly your taste buds will adapt to less sugar in your food. I have included some sugar-free desserts at the back of this book.

Seaweed/sea vegetables

The name seaweed is rather off-putting and so I prefer to use the term sea vegetables, which is actually more accurate. Sea vegetables are sold dried in packets in health food shops, along with some lovely seaweed snacks. These are low in calories, fat free and provide an excellent source of iodine (which regulates your metabolism).

They're also a decent source of calcium, zinc, manganese, chromium and selenium.

Good sea vegetables to try to include: dulse, kombu (a Japanese form of kelp), wakame, agar, nori, arame and hiziki.

Sea vegetables can be used in a number of different ways, for example in soups, salads, sushi and other savoury dishes.

A valid concern regarding eating sea vegetables is that, because they are harvested from the sea, they could be laden with pollutants such as lead, cadmium and mercury. However, if you buy from a reputable company you can be assured that the sea vegetables are grown in clear water away from known areas of pollution. After harvesting, the sea vegetables are also tested independently for heavy metal contamination.

• Chapter 5 •

Still Can't Lose Weight?

You're eating all the right foods. You're making sure your blood sugar levels are kept steady by eating every three hours. You're exercising. You're not giving in to crazy binges or inappropriate snacks. And yet you *still* aren't losing weight. The vast majority of people will find that, by following my simple guidelines, they will lose weight easily and effortlessly, slowly and naturally. But there are some people who will need a little extra help. This chapter looks at why sometimes weight won't shift and, more importantly, what you can do about it.

It could be your thyroid

Many people have an underactive thyroid which can contribute to weight gain and this is more common in women. This is something you will need to ask your doctor to check for you, with a blood test. But this simple questionnaire will give you a good idea if it might be an issue for you. If you answer 'yes' to four or more of the following questions, your thyroid could be underactive and you should head to your GP.

- Has your weight gone up gradually over months for no apparent reason?
- Do you feel the cold more than most?
- Are you often constipated?
- Are you often depressed, forgetful or confused?
- Are you losing hair or is it drier than it used to be?
- Is your skin drier than it used to be?
- Are you having menstrual problems?
- Are you having difficulty falling pregnant?
- Have you noticed a lack of energy?
- Are you getting headaches?

Your thyroid gland is situated in your neck. Along with the hypothalamus and pituitary glands in your brain, it helps control your metabolism. It produces two hormones, thyroxine and triiodothyronine, production of which is triggered by the hypothalamus and the pituitary, which also produce thyrotropin-releasing hormone and thyroid-stimulating hormone (TSH). Underactive or hypothyroidism is a deficiency (lack) of thyroid hormone, caused by either failure of the pituitary gland to produce TSH or failure of the thyroid itself.

It is estimated that there are over one hundred symptoms of thyroid imbalance and, because of this huge range, it can often be difficult to diagnose. The symptoms of an underactive thyroid can also mimic other problems so it may take your doctor some time to sort out the real problem and prescribe the correct treatment. However, there is a blood test available to assess thyroid function and, if you think you have a problem, you should ask your doctor for this test.

Unfortunately, mild forms of underactivity can go undetected by the test so your doctor may not offer medication to assist you. From a medical point of view, the test will show that your thyroid is functioning within the normal range. However, this does not cancel out the possibility that even a mild thyroid underactivity could be affecting your weight.

Before you despair, there is another way to test your thyroid function.

The most popular way of testing thyroid function, before the advent of the blood test, was to measure basal body temperature. Even if you haven't considered that your thyroid might be underactive it could be worth doing this test at home.

Basal means your body's temperature at rest. If the temperature is too low it may indicate that you have a sluggish metabolism caused by an underactive thyroid.

You need to take your temperature once a day for three days. Women should do this test on the second, third and fourth days of the menstrual cycle. The female body temperature rises after ovulation so it wouldn't give a clear picture if done later in the cycle. Non-menstruating women and men should take their temperature on any three consecutive days. Basal body temperature should read between 36.4 and 36.7 degrees C (97.6 and 98.2 degrees F).

How to measure your basal body temperature

- You will need a thermometer. (The traditional type is fine but there are some good electronic ones on the market which only take a minute to register the temperature and bleep when it is done.)
- Put the thermometer by your bed before you go to sleep.
- On waking, remain lying in bed – do not have a drink or walk to the bathroom before you take your temperature. Put the thermometer under your armpit and leave it there until it bleeps. If you are using the traditional type leave if for 10 minutes, having made sure the mercury was as its lowest point before you began.
- Make a note of your temperature on each of the three mornings and calculate your average temperature.

If your average falls below 35.6 degrees C (97.6 degrees F) then your thyroid may not be functioning properly.

If you have already had the blood test done and the result was normal but your average temperature is low, then you would need to look at natural remedies to help improve thyroid function. My clinic would be happy to help (either in person or by phone or Skype, see the back of this book for contact details).

You're leaving too long between meals

Your metabolic rate increases during digestion of food – this is called the thermal effect of food. That is why it is important to eat little and often. Remember that even after just five hours without food, your body starts to believe it is being starved and will decrease your metabolism. So if, after seven or eight hours of sleep, you then miss breakfast, you are putting your body into fasting mode and you are more likely to store fat, rather than use it.

Your brown fat may not be active enough (blame that thyroid again)

You *need* body fat. It insulates you from the cold and keeps your skin and arteries supple. There are two kinds of fat cells, brown and white (sometimes called yellow). Brown fat is darker as it contains a large number of mitochondria (power houses) which are portions of cells where energy is made and burned off. Because brown fat has a large number of mitochondria it means that is very metabolically active and a great deal of energy is burned. White fat is not so active and it stores energy and produces hormones. It is this fat that tends to accumulate in various parts of our body, especially on women, and especially around the hips, abdomen, thighs and buttocks. Brown fat tends to be situated deeper inside the body.

The ability of brown fat to produce heat is called thermogenesis. As you eat more calories, the brown fat balances the intake by converting fat into heat and so burning more fat. If the brown fat is fairly active you will be less likely to store white fat. Slim people seem to possess the most effective brown fat heat-producing ability, whereas people who gain weight don't seem to be so good at it.

Thermogenesis can be stimulated by thyroid hormone. So, when your thyroid is working efficiently, you are usually warm and have warm hands and feet. When it isn't you feel the cold. That is why it is well worth taking your body temperature as described earlier in this chapter to see whether your body temperature is too low.

It could be your prescribed drugs

Weight gain is often linked to certain medications such as hormone replacement therapy (HRT), the contraceptive pill and steroids. Some anti-depressants can also cause increased appetite and weight gain. If you have to take medication, discuss your weight problem with your doctor and ask if there are alternative drugs you could take. On no account should you stop taking medication without guidance from your doctor.

It may be a food intolerance

The term 'food allergy' is used to describe a specific response by the immune system to a substance (inhaled, touched or eaten) that it mistakenly identifies as harmful. The response can be immediate. Common foods that are linked to this type of allergy are shellfish, strawberries and, more severely, peanuts. Symptoms can range from a rash to a slight fever to, more unpleasantly, diarrhoea or constipation. In extreme cases, the allergy can cause a serious reaction which can close up the airways and this requires urgent medical attention. This is known as anaphylactic shock and can be fatal.

There are other, less dramatic, types of reactions to food called food intolerances. With these reactions there can be a delay in the onset of the symptoms (from four to 72 hours), and the foods are often eaten in larger amounts and more frequently. They don't cause acute illness and seldom are they bad enough to warrant a visit to the doctor, yet they can generate regular minor symptoms which are often uncomfortable. These symptoms can include bloating, diarrhoea, constipation and flatulence, lethargy, arthritis, fatigue, skin problems, eczema, joint and muscle pains, stuffy nose, recurrent infections, anxiety, depression, insomnia, irritability, water retention, headaches, migraines and, you guessed it, weight gain.

If you suspect a food intolerance and want to confirm it, you can either have a blood test (this is explained fully in Chapter 8) or try an elimination diet for two weeks.

The two food groups which cause most of the problems are gluten grains (wheat, rye and barley) and dairy products (cow, sheep and goat products including butter, cheese, milk and yogurt), so it would be worth excluding these for two weeks along with caffeinated drinks (tea, coffee, colas), alcohol and artificial additives (such as artificial sweeteners, colourings, preservatives and flavourings).

Be organised so that you are well stocked with the foods you are allowed. Try to follow this plan at a time when you have some degree of control over your meals and not too many social events pending. Eat when you need and don't feel deprived. Keep it up for two weeks if you possibly can, although you may still get good results if you can only follow the regime for a week.

You must persevere during the first few days. You may feel slightly unwell as your body experiences withdrawal symptoms from certain stimulants such as tea and coffee. You may even develop flu-like symptoms such as headaches, general aches and pains and even diarrhoea. But the result is worth the discomfort – most people find their energy has increased after completing the exclusion diet. This is not surprising as their body is no longer diverting energy to battle with foods that don't agree with it.

You will have to do a bit of label reading because one of the gluten grains – wheat – can be found in many surprising foods; not just the usual bread, pasta, biscuits and cakes. Wheat can be used in sausages as a filler, as a thickener in sauces, in soups, gravy and stock cubes and soya sauce (wheat-free soya sauce is known as tamari). Dairy foods can be found in breakfast cereals, chocolate, bread and processed meats – watch out if the label says lactose or whey.

If you feel better after the two weeks, the next step is food challenging – you begin by adding back one food (and only one food) at a time. So, maybe, start with adding back cow's milk. Keep a simple food and symptom diary so that you can make a note of how you feel. Do you feel bloated or tired? Do you have joint pains? Have other symptoms returned?

If you notice a return of old symptoms then you have at least one culprit. Unfortunately, you may find you have more than one intolerance, so you will need to be patient and challenge each individual food, one at a time. It *is* time-consuming but it's well worth it so do take the time and make the effort. Allow everything to settle down (leave at least two days in between testing foods because the reaction may be slower than you think because of the journey time through your digestive system). Now test something else – say, wheat – and repeat the process. It can be quite an eye-opener.

Once you have a clear idea of what you are reacting to, it's up to you whether or not to re-introduce certain foods. Say wheat is a problem and you realise it is making you retain weight, you may decide to eliminate it until you are down to a comfortable size. You could then gradually re-introduce wheat, perhaps one slice of toast a day or a portion of pasta and see whether you feel any differently. Having an intolerance is not necessarily a life sentence. Most of the time we eat too much of the foods that disagree with us and so can overload our bodies. Once your body has recovered from the overload, you may find you can tolerate some foods if you eat them in moderation.

Could it be *Candida*?

So, you've looked at your thyroid and it's fine. You've worked through possible food intolerances and they don't seem to be your problem. Don't despair. There is one other factor that's worth considering: *Candida.*

Do you get any of these symptoms?

- Sugar cravings
- Cravings for foods such as wine, bread, cheese
- Migraines or headaches
- Chronic thrush (yeast infection)
- Inability to lose weight
- You feel tired all the time
- You wake up feeling tired even after eight hours' sleep
- You often feel spaced out
- You feel drunk on even a small amount of alcohol
- You have a bloated, even swollen abdomen and excess flatulence

If several of these apply then you may have a *Candida albicans* overgrowth. We all have the yeast *Candida albicans* in our gut, skin and in the vagina but it is usually controlled by beneficial bacteria. When the immune system is compromised, say because of illness or bad diet, the *Candida* can grow out of control.

This overgrowth can also be caused by antibiotics, use of the contraceptive pill, HRT, steroids and stress – all of which can reduce the beneficial bacteria that normally controls the *Candida*.

There is a simple, at home test for *Candida* overgrowth. If you do find out you have a *Candida* problem you will need to go on an anti-*Candida* diet (to stop feeding the yeast), take probiotics (to increase the levels of beneficial bacteria) and also take food supplements to help eliminate the *Candida* overgrowth. Don't worry – in Chapter 8 I give all the details on testing for *Candida* and then how to tackle the problem.

Chapter 6

Get Moving – Why Exercise Matters

It's a modern-day puzzle – we eat fewer calories than we did a hundred years ago and yet we are getting fatter rather than thinner. Why? It can be attributed to many factors, such as changes in the type of food we eat, but one of the main reasons is that, nowadays, we're far more sedentary.

Our ancestors didn't have to 'exercise' – being active was part of their everyday life. Even recently, people thought nothing of walking a few miles to and from work or school. Every household chore required a good deal of effort and was physically demanding: for example, the weekly wash was done by hand and involved a lot of scrubbing and wringing. In stark contrast nowadays, we drive the car to and from the shops, we put the family's clothes in the washing machine and, as for housework, we have endless gadgets to make life easier. Our lives are increasingly spent at screens, which usually means sitting for long periods – at desks at work or on the sofa at home. Most of us would agree that life is less physically demanding now than it has been for previous generations. The downside of this is that few of us actually get the exercise our bodies truly need.

Exercise seems to have become a luxury – something with which to pamper yourself. Just as you might treat yourself to a new hairstyle or a manicure you might indulge yourself with membership of a smart gym.

All of us need to make exercise a conscious part of our lives but it doesn't have to be an expensive luxury. We don't have to join expensive fitness centres or go to trendy classes.

Instead, you could do what people did in the past and incorporate activity into everyday life:

- Choose to walk up stairs instead of taking the lift.
- Walk up escalators.
- Run, rather than walk, up the stairs at home.
- Park the car or get off the bus further away from work or the shops.
- Use a standing desk.

- Pace rather than sit or stand still when on the phone.
- Meet friends for a walk or jog rather than a sit down in a café.

None of us would want to go back to the days when household jobs were an endless, demoralising grind of exhausting physical effort but we all have to find some ways of making up for the lack of everyday exercise in our lives.

Why exercise?

The benefits of regular exercise cannot be exaggerated. The older we get, the more important exercise is for our health. Regular exercise has been linked to a lower risk of cancer, dementia, type 2 diabetes, depression, heart disease and a higher tolerance to stress. The World Health Organization (WHO) recommends we all get at least 150 minutes of exercise a week and that's not even for fitness gains, that's for our general health[68]. Do you want to gain and keep a youthful figure? Have great skin, a better sex life and more energy? Do you want to kick out stress and feel calmer and brighter? Do you want to have a real zest for life? Exercise is the answer.

Exercise can have a powerful all-round effect on your health. Apart from the feelings of wellbeing it brings (it's a proven antidepressant), there are physical benefits you might not have considered. Moderate exercise performed at a time of day other than just before bed helps improve sleep quality and can also soothe insomnia. Exercise helps to keep your bowels working efficiently, which means you are eliminating waste products your body doesn't need, and it helps keep your gut microbes diverse and plentiful. It also improves the function of your immune system, your lymph system and the ability of your body to keep blood sugar in balance. It stimulates thyroid gland hormone production and helps to improve thyroid function which has a direct effect on your metabolism. This is especially important if you have an underactive thyroid (see Chapter 5). So it's definitely worth getting moving!

Metabolism and exercise

We are all governed by our metabolic rate which is exclusive to us. That's why some eating plans might work for a friend but not for you. Understanding and getting to know your metabolism can help you with weight loss and maintenance.

An athletic person who has a high ratio of muscle to fat will have a higher metabolic rate than a person of the same weight with a lower muscle to fat ratio. This is because it takes more calories to maintain muscle tissue than fat tissue so the higher muscle to fat ratio athlete will be able to eat more calories than the lower ratio person without gaining weight.

Some people are fortunate enough to be born with a metabolism that causes them little trouble, but others aren't. There are times in most slimmers' lives when their metabolism becomes the enemy within. Exercise can help because it boosts your metabolism and allows you to burn fat more efficiently. This means that you are burning off fat and calories at a faster rate than if you did no exercise. Research has shown that your metabolic rate can remain higher for at least 15 hours after exercising.

The human body is very good at adapting to what we ask it to do though. So once it gets used to that 30 minute walk, for example, it will not need to burn as many calories to do it. That's why it's important to keep building on and changing the activities you do as you get fitter. This will prevent a weight-loss plateau and keep your metabolism fired.

What is the best exercise for weight loss?

Ideas on the best exercise for weight loss have changed dramatically over the years. It is now thought that a combination of both aerobic and resistance training gives the best fat loss and best inch loss, and has the most beneficial effect on blood sugar levels[69].

In order to lose weight, you want to build muscle. The more muscle you have the more fat you burn (even at rest)".

Because muscle weighs more than fat, it can be misleading to weigh yourself or calculate your BMI (as previously discussed) when you start on a weight loss/exercise regime. You either need to measure your body fat percentage or use a tape measure and monitor inch loss. Muscle takes up five times less space than fat so you will look and feel slimmer even if your weight remains the same or even increases.

Over the past few years, the concept of high-intensity interval training (HIIT) has come to the fore. This suggests that we could gain significant benefits (predominantly fat burning and blood sugar balance) by doing short bursts of intense exercise, rather than long sessions of steady-state exercise.

We know that with regular steady-state cardiovascular exercise your body will only start to burn your fat stores once you have been exercising for 20 minutes. Before that it takes energy from your muscles. Thirty minutes jogging on a treadmill burns about 200 calories – the equivalent of two cappuccinos (without added sugar), two glasses of wine or half a muffin.

So to exercise in a way that promotes weight loss, it is better to do a combination of two activities:

1. High-intensity interval training.
2. Resistance training to build muscle.

High-intensity interval training (HIIT)

With HIIT you try and work at your maximum for a short burst of time (30 to 60 seconds) and then reduce the level to a moderate pace (even walking) and then go back to the high intensity again. This is repeated a number of times. There are many variations of HIIT and your choice should depend on how fit you are. If you have not exercised for a long time, then you would need to take this gradually. Some HIIT sessions can last for as short a time as four minutes and others up to 30 minutes. This means that even if lack of time was always a limiting factor in exercising, then HIIT is a way round this while still getting good results.

One of the most popular high intensity trainings is Tabata training, created by Dr Izumi Tabata from Japan. The whole protocol only lasts for four minutes (not including a warm up and cool down) but it can produce remarkable results:

- Five minutes' warm up.
- High-intensity activity for 20 seconds.
- Rest for 10 seconds.
- Repeat this eight times (takes four minutes in total).
- Two minutes' cool down.

This type of interval training has been shown to be more effective at helping you to lose weight than long cardiovascular workouts. Your body will burn more fat when the intensity is higher and weight loss continues after the exercise has finished. Those four minutes of interval training are more effective than one hour of steady aerobic exercise because it shocks your body into taking energy from your fat stores rather than using energy from your muscles.

The other good thing about HITT is that it works for any kind of exercise where you can vary the intensity. Use an exercise bike, a cross trainer or a rowing machine or even running or power walking in the park, and aim for three of these short sessions a week.

Resistance training

Resistance or strength training helps you to build muscle, which then helps you to burn fat and lose those inches. The same WHO recommendations on exercise suggests we all need to incorporate strength training twice a week[70]. You can use dumbbells, weight machines in the gym, kettlebells, bands, or you can just use your own body weight (triceps dips, squats, lunges, pull-ups, planks, press ups and so on). You can modify all the exercises to suit your ability – for example, you can do a box press-up on your knees if a full press-up is too challenging.

Why resistance training? It breaks down muscle fibres which then, during the rest period between sessions, is able to rebuild stronger and better. This is why fitness instructors will advise that you train different muscle groups in each session (say, upper body in one session and then lower body in the next). It's also important that you give your muscles the chance to recover and repair in between sessions. So don't exercise the same muscle groups each day. Any weight-bearing exercise is also valuable for building and maintaining bone, which is especially important for women as we age, to keep osteoporosis at bay.

When you start using weights, start small. Begin with a light weight and build up slowly. You should be aiming for three sets of repetitions. So, you will aim to lift the weight 12 times, then rest for a minute and repeat. Do this three times. Lift the weights slowly and mindfully, maintaining good posture and a strong core. Use your breath, breathing out with the effort of lifting, and breathing in as you slowly and smoothly return the weight. You will soon realise if the weight is at the right level. If it's too light, you will find you could easily go beyond your 12 repetitions. If it's too heavy, you will struggle to get to six. Ideally, your muscles should be tiring by your third set – and you will only be able to get to around eight or 10 repetitions. Once you're easily reaching 12 repetitions on the third set, then it's time to increase the weight size or resistance.

For resistance exercises you can perform in the gym and at home see the following pages.

A Good Resistance Programme

This set of six exercises (continued over the page) will help you to burn off fat because weight training increases your metabolism. Use a set of dumbells for each exercise (or you could use rice-, or sand-filled bags or even a couple of food cans or bottles of water). Do a number of repetitions (e.g. 12) for each exercise and then rest for two or three minutes before repeating the set two more times.

Take great care to do the exercises properly rather than fighting with weights that are too heavy. When using weights for the first time, always use the lightest weights available.

Exercise 1: **Lateral rise**

The arms should be raised only to shoulder level and the elbows kept bent to take the load off the elbow joint.

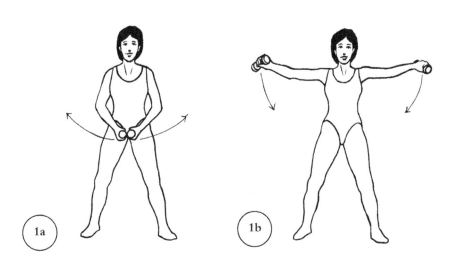

Exercise 2: **Alternate arm raise**

Raise each arm alternately in front of the body while keeping the elbows and knees slightly bent. Take care not to arch your back.

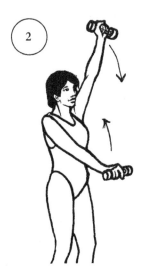

Exercise 3: **Curls**

These can be done in either the seated or standing position and with arms together or alternately.

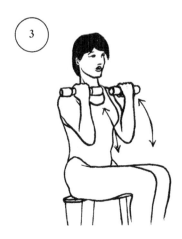

Exercise 4: **Abdominal crunch**

Lie on your back with your knees raised. While doing the crunches keep the lower back supported on the floor, don't arch your back. Aim the dumbells towards the knees during the lift.

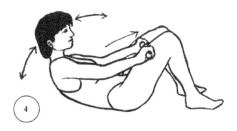

Exercise 5: **Abdominal crunch through the legs**

Lie on your back with your legs raised in the air and wide apart. Pass the dumbells through your open legs.

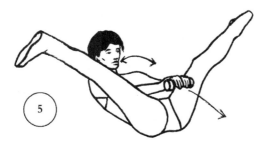

Exercise 6: **One arm bent**

On your knees, supporting your body by resting on one arm on the floor, slightly in front of your shoulders. Pull the weight to the shoulder without arching your back. Repeat both sides.

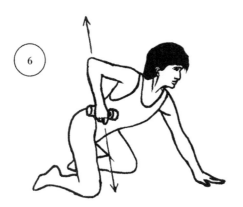

If you join a gym you will be given an induction by a fitness instructor who should find out your goals and put together a programme that will help you reach them. He or she should also show you how to use each piece of equipment safely. If you are unsure at all, it is imperative that you ask for help. If you do not follow correct technique you could, at best, fail to reach your fitness potential and, at worst, injure yourself.

Exercise tips

- If you can, time your exercise so you're working on an empty stomach. The ideal time is before breakfast because you will burn more fat and this will help you to become more insulin sensitive.

- Many people like to separate their cardio sessions and weight-training sessions. But if you're short on time and need to combine both in the same session, then always do the weight training first. Have a five-minute aerobic warm up (cycling, rowing, cross trainer, treadmill fast walking) then move straight into weight training. This is important as it means you won't be too tired when you come to the weight-training session. Also, you will burn more fat during your cardio session because you will have used up the energy in your muscles.

- Always have protein (even if it's just a snack) within half an hour of exercise to help with muscle repair and growth. Either time your training so you can have breakfast afterwards or have a snack – meat, eggs, fish, nuts, seeds. Or try a protein shake (hemp or pea protein are good sources of protein, mix with nut milk and add a banana for flavour).

- Make sure you're always well-hydrated. Drinking water is essential to weight loss, because fat burning increases levels of toxins in your system. These will then need to be flushed out by your liver and kidneys. If you don't drink enough water, your body will burn fat less efficiently.

- Don't exercise every day. Once you get into exercise it can tempting as it feels so good, but the body needs rest days. If you don't have the chance to recuperate between exercise sessions, you can actually lose muscle. Then your metabolism will slow down, so you are solving nothing. Let your body recover properly, then you will be able to work at maximum capacity in your next workout and burn yet more fat.

Once you build up a solid exercise programme and keep to it, you will swiftly notice differences in how you look. Although it's tempting to peek, try to keep away from the scales. Muscle weighs more than fat, so you might well find you are actually putting on pounds initially – but this is good! What you're aiming for is to build muscle and lose fat – ignore the scales and focus on how your clothes feel and, even more importantly, how *you* feel in yourself.

Keep going – studies show that, if you can maintain a new regime for six weeks, you will have built a really healthy habit and will find it much easier to continue. You will also notice that, not only are you feeling fitter and looking better, your mood will be improving. This, in turn, will strengthen your resolve when it comes to the eating part of your weight-loss life plan. Above all, be patient with yourself. If you keep eating healthily, exercising regularly and enjoying your life, your body will eventually settle at a weight that is perfect for you.

Fat burning and metabolism

As we've already seen, exercise allows you to burn fat more efficiently. It boosts your metabolism so that you burn off fat at a faster rate even after you've stopped exercising.

All forms of activity are beneficial for your health, so keep up the walks in the park and anything else you enjoy that gets you moving. But for losing weight you need to try something different and add in the HIIT and resistance training. You won't regret it.

MORE REASONS TO GET MOVING:

Exercise soothes your emotions

Exercise releases brain chemicals called endorphins, which helps you to feel happier, more alert and calmer. These have a dramatically positive effect on people suffering from depression, stress, anxiety and insomnia, and exercise is often recommended as part of the treatment for these problems.

Therefore, if you know that you are prone to overeating when you are stressed, anxious or depressed, use exercise to change your mood and lift yourself out of this vicious cycle.

Exercise fuels your love life

When you are full of energy and vitality you will be much more interested in sex. Perhaps sometimes you feel you are just too tired to make love but by doing exercise you will find that your sex life will be re-energised – all you've got to do is make that initial effort and find the energy to exercise. Once the right chemicals start flowing, so will romance!

Holidays are a good example. You relax from the normal pressures, you swim, walk, maybe go dancing and suddenly you find you have energy for things you would be far too tired for at home – including sex. Why wait for a holiday for this to happen? Get yourself fit and active so that you'll enjoy making love regularly. The combination of exercise and good eating will help you to lose weight, making you much more confident about your body, which will also help your love life.

Sex itself could be classed as a form of exercise, as it increases your heart rate and it has been estimated to have the equivalent benefit of a good run.

Exercise helps your heart

Exercise increases your circulation and also lowers LDL (the 'bad') cholesterol and increases HDL (the 'good') cholesterol. Regular exercise can help to reduce blood pressure, one of the main risk factors for heart disease, and is especially good for varicose veins.

Exercise protects against cancer

The World Cancer Research Fund has found evidence that exercise helps protect against bowel cancer, womb (endometrial) cancer and breast cancer. It is thought that physical activity strengthens your immune system and this can help protect you against abnormal cell growth.

One study showed that women who exercise for around four hours a week have a 58 per cent lower risk of breast cancer and that those who routinely exercised for between one and three hours a week had a 30 per cent lower risk[71]. Other research has shown that all types of exercise, even household activities, reduce the risk of breast cancer so the message is clear: we need to keep active to protect our health[72].

It is thought that regular exercise modifies a woman's hormonal activity in a beneficial way. We know that extremes of exercise alter the menstrual cycle dramatically – many athletes and ballet dancers, for instance, don't have periods at all. The suggestion, therefore, is that moderate, routine exercise suppresses the overproduction of female hormones, which reduces a woman's exposure to them during her lifetime.

Exercise is a stress reliever

Normally when the stress hormones are released your life is in danger and your body expects you to run or fight. But with our modern lifestyles of traffic jams, missed appointments, work and family upsets, the same hormones are released but there is no physical action (you could just be sitting and seething). When you exercise you are giving your body that physical outlet. You're 'letting off steam' and so reducing the impact of the stress hormones on your health.

Exercise is vital for your bones

Astronauts lose bone density in the weightlessness of space because no demands are put on their bones. The same principle applies to the rest of us – if we don't make demands on our bones they will weaken. This is true for both sexes but particularly for women as they go through the menopause and face the risk of osteoporosis.

The key really is 'use it, don't lose it'. If you make demands on your body and bones then your bone density will be maintained or increased. Achieve this by making sure your life contains a fair amount of physical exercise, either through your regular lifestyle or via organised exercise.

When your bones are put under pressure via weight bearing exercise, your body will build stronger bone. If you are inactive and make no demands on your bones, you will, over time, compromise your bone health.

The impact of exercise has been dramatically illustrated by research that examined the difference between the two arms of professional tennis players. The bones of the racket-holding arm, which does most of the work, can be over one third denser than those of the other arm.

But don't worry if tennis isn't your game! Other forms of weight-bearing exercise that puts demands on your bones include:

- Resistance training
- Brisk walking
- Running
- Circuit training/bootcamp workouts
- Aerobics
- Dancing
- Badminton

And don't forget everyday activities such as:

- Stair climbing
- Housework
- Shopping (just not on the internet!)
- Gardening
- Decorating and DIY

Any physical exercise is better than none. Couch potatoes don't just gain weight, they also allow their bone density to drain away. We all become more frail as we age and some loss of bone density is inevitable. However, through exercise you can keep this loss to a minimum. Women should be especially careful about bone density because their risk of osteoporosis and fractures increases later in life.

Exercise can help women maintain or even increase their bone density through and beyond the menopause.

Exercise maintains mobility

Exercise keeps our reflexes sharp, joints well oiled, muscles and tendons strong and flexible, and improves balance and co-ordination. All these factors become more important as you pass the age of 40. As we get older, our range of movement automatically becomes more limited unless we make the effort through exercise to maintain it. Stumbles, falls and misjudged steps can all too easily and quickly lead to injuries which might never have happened if we had kept ourselves physically active and agile.

Can you do too much exercise?

The simple answer is yes. Too much exercise can cause a change in the body-fat ratio and in women can stop periods. Very young female gymnasts and athletes have found that over-exercising has prevented their periods from even starting at all. Most of us, of course, come nowhere near to over-exercising but some people can become addicted to exercise, very often those who have had eating problems when they were younger.

It's also possible to exercise too hard and risk burn out. People who train for endurance events like marathons and ultra-marathons, triathlons and cycling events – all of which are becoming more popular – can overtrain and this can lead to injury and illness, as their immune systems are compromised. This is easily avoided if you remember that rest days, relaxation, good nutrition and hydration are key to a healthy exercise regime.

The vast majority of us, though, particularly those seeking to lose weight, don't need to worry about exercising too much because we're not doing enough.

How to design your own exercise programme

As regular exercise is more beneficial than occasional bursts, it is best to find something you enjoy which will motivate you to do it regularly. Brisk walking is a great choice as it can be fitted in at any time. It does not require any special equipment or clothing and costs nothing. As well as being beneficial for you physically, it also frees your mind so that your imagination can just 'wander off' while you walk. This can help to alleviate stress. If you have not exercised for years, walking is a good way to start getting fit.

Don't rush out on to the tennis court if you haven't played for years, or suddenly begin a really tough cardiovascular sport or exercise programme if you know you are even a little unfit. It's a sure recipe for a nasty muscle injury or even worse. If you have not been exercising regularly, take things slowly at first and build up gradually. Aim to do a little more this week than you did last week. If you have any health concerns always consult your doctor before starting exercise.

Choose an exercise that fits in with your lifestyle

How we exercise is very much a matter of personal choice. We are all individuals so we have to find an exercise routine that fits in with our families, our lifestyle and our finances. Some people will prefer to exercise on their own, others need the motivation of a group or a friend to keep them going. Use whatever way suits you best so you are more likely to keep active and fit in the long term.

Make health your goal

You will find, as many others have done, that on the road to becoming fit and enjoying the pleasures of food, you will automatically lose weight and fat. If you make health your goal rather than focusing on losing weight, your whole perspective on food will change. You'll find you achieve your appropriate weight without having to go on endless diets.

Chapter 7

Supplements to Help with Weight Loss

The food and exercise guidelines I've already covered will, without doubt, allow you to lose weight healthily and naturally. There are, however, a few more things you can do to help reach your happy weight and shape. Nutritional supplements can be helpful in improving metabolism, maintaining a stable appetite, eliminating cravings, detoxifying your body and generally getting you back into good health by restoring balance throughout your body. They're the only 'diet pills' you should even think about trying!

Food is, and should be regarded as, a powerful medicine – it has a huge impact on the biochemical processes of your body. Good nutrition is not just about eating well but also about correcting any vitamin or mineral deficiencies. You need to eat a good variety of food to give your body the best possible chance of getting all the nutrients it needs.

Vitamins and minerals work in harmony; most of them are dependent on each other to work efficiently. The best way to structure a supplement programme for yourself is to take a good multivitamin and mineral supplement. You can then add in other supplements that might be useful.

A number of chemical reactions are involved in turning glucose into energy instead of fat. These are controlled by enzymes, which are themselves dependent on vitamins and minerals in the body. If any of these are deficient, you will find you lack energy, you feel low and, when it comes to weight loss, you will find your body stores glucose as fat instead of turning it into energy. So it can be helpful to top up your body with these vitamins and minerals. There are also some nutrients which are extremely helpful in getting rid of that extra weight while you are sorting out your new eating plan and exercise programme. Remember, these are not a substitute for eating well; as the name suggests they are *supplementary* to your food.

If you have been yo-yo dieting, either restricting food intake or trying different diet drinks or pills, it is likely that you are deficient in a number of vitamins and minerals. Supplements could certainly help if you know you've been depriving yourself for a long time, possibly even years. Nowadays, a lot of our food is refined and, therefore, stripped of valuable nutrients – even the soil our food grows in is depleted of nutrients through overuse.

When it comes to buying supplements you do get what you pay for. I would recommend buying capsules rather than tablets, as tablets will contain binding agents to hold the nutrients together. Binding agents can include sucrose, lactose, sugar alcohols like sorbitol or synthetic polymers such as polyethylene glycol, none of which are ideal when you are 'cleaning' up your food.

Choose capsules that are only filled with the active ingredients, as some capsules can contain excipients (inert substances combined with the nutrients) such as anti-caking agents. These are added purely for the manufacturers' benefit as they help the nutrients flow more easily through the filling process. They do absolutely nothing for you. Once again, it comes down to reading the labels. I use a number of different supplement companies in my clinics and I have formulated a range of supplements for The Natural Health Practice (NHP) which are all capsules and don't contain any excipients at all (see www.naturalhealthpractice.com).

Why vitamins?

Vitamins are essential for life and are required in small amounts for healthy growth and development. Your body is unable to make many of them itself, so it is vital that you obtain them either from the food you eat or in supplement form.

The B vitamins are often called the 'stress' vitamins because of their ability to help you cope with the pressures of everyday life. Vitamins B3 and B6 are especially important as they help to supply fuel to cells, ready for burning for energy. Vitamin B6 is necessary, together with zinc, for the production of pancreatic enzymes which help the effective digestion of food. If your digestion is good then you will efficiently use up your food instead of storing it as fat.

Vitamins B2, B3 and B6 are necessary for normal thyroid hormone production, so any deficiencies in these can affect thyroid function and consequently affect your metabolism. Vitamin B3 is also a component of the glucose tolerance factor (GTF), which is released every time your blood sugar rises.

Vitamin B5 plays an important role in energy production and is also necessary for optimum adrenal function.

Vitamin C is important for your immune function and research has also shown that if you have good levels of vitamin C when you exercise you will burn off 30 per cent more fat than if you had low levels of vitamin C. Also when you are under stress, your body uses more vitamin C so it is important to have good levels[73].

Vitamins that help weight loss and where to find them:

Vitamin B1

Function: Important for energy production, nervous system support.

Good food sources: Beans, wholegrains, nuts, seeds, green leafy vegetables.

Vitamin B2

Function: Releases energy from carbohydrates. Turns fat, sugar and protein into energy. Needed for healthy hair, nails and eyes.

Good food sources: Eggs, green leafy vegetables, seaweeds, soya beans, peas, sardines, mackerel, yogurt.

Vitamin B3

Function: Needed for energy production. Balances blood sugar. Controls cholesterol.

Good food sources: Tuna in oil, salmon, wholewheat products, asparagus, almonds, brown rice.

Vitamin B5

Function: Used in the utilisation of fats, carbohydrates and proteins as energy sources. Important for hormone production and healthy adrenal function.

Good food sources: Wholegrains, yogurt, peas, lentils, eggs, mushrooms, brown rice.

Vitamin B6

Function: Helps with carbohydrate metabolism. Important in maintaining hormone balance. Useful for PMS and depression.

Good food sources: Tuna, salmon, wholegrains, cauliflower, herring, soya, sweet potatoes, sunflower seeds.

Vitamin C

Function: Needed to make collagen for healthy bones, skin, muscles and joints. Critical to immune function and an important antioxidant. Turns food into energy.

Good food sources: Raw pepper, broccoli, cauliflower, strawberries, peas, oranges.

Minerals

Minerals contained in the soil are absorbed by plants and, in turn, we eat those plants and ingest the minerals. Unfortunately, over time, our soil has been depleted of some of the minerals, through over-farming and the use of pesticides, and so there are now far fewer minerals in the plants we eat than a couple of generations ago. Compared to the 1930s, the fruits and vegetables we eat contain an average of 20 per cent fewer minerals. Magnesium has been depleted by 24 per cent, calcium by 46 per cent, iron by 27 per cent and zinc by 59 per cent.

With regard to meat and dairy, iron in meat has been depleted by 47 per cent, iron in milk by over 60 per cent, calcium loss in cheese by 15 per cent and Parmesan cheese by 70 per cent[74].

Also our fruit and vegetables can be flown hundreds of miles and can sit in a warehouse for a period of time before getting to the shelves, causing nutrients to be reduced.

Mineral supplements like calcium should be taken in the form of citrates or ascorbates which are more easily absorbed by the body. Sulphates, carbonates and oxides are inorganic forms of the minerals and should be avoided, since they are not so easily assimilated: mineral supplements in this form may pass through the body without being absorbed. For instance, you can absorb 30 per cent more calcium from a calcium citrate supplement than from a calcium carbonate supplement[75]. Calcium carbonate is literally chalk, it is mined from the ground and we do not eat calcium in that form, but it is cheap for the manufacturers. Once again, read those labels!

Minerals that help weight loss and where to find them:

Zinc

Function: Zinc is an important mineral for appetite control and a deficiency of zinc can cause a loss of taste and smell so that you crave and seek stronger tasting food including more salty, sugary and/or spicy foods. Zinc also functions together with vitamins A and E in the manufacture of thyroid hormone. Zinc is necessary for the correct action of many hormones including leptin, which is produced by fat cells and controls appetite and hunger, and insulin, so important in balancing blood sugar. It's also important for fertility in both men and women.

Good food sources: Oysters, pumpkin seeds, wholegrains, almonds, peas.

Chromium

Function: Chromium has been the most widely-researched mineral with regard to its effectiveness as an aid to weight loss. It helps to control cravings and binge eating by maintaining blood sugar balance and reducing hunger. Chromium is needed for the metabolism of sugar and without it insulin is less effective in controlling blood sugar levels. It is the major nutrient in glucose tolerance factor (GTF). It also helps to control levels of fat and cholesterol in the blood.

Good food sources: Wholegrains, apples, eggs, parsnips, carrots.

Magnesium

Function: Magnesium is known as 'nature's tranquilliser' and is especially important if you are under stress, as stress can push you to eat unhealthily. Magnesium also helps balance your blood sugar by helping with the production and action of insulin. In addition, it is an important mineral for your bone health, muscle relaxation and recovery, sleep, energy and for lowering blood pressure.

Good food sources: Wholegrains, pumpkin seeds, soya.

Manganese

Function: Manganese helps with the metabolism of fats and also helps to stabilise blood sugar. It functions in many enzyme systems in your body, including the enzymes involved in energy metabolism and thyroid hormone function.

Good food sources: Almonds, wholegrains, Brussels sprouts, carrots.

Other useful nutrients for weight loss

It's not just vitamins and minerals that are useful for helping us in our weight loss goal. There are other some other supplements that are worth considering. Let's look at the most beneficial.

Co-Enzyme Q10

Co-Enzyme Q10 is important for energy production. It's found in all the tissues and organs of our bodies and, as we get older, we may become deficient, which can results in a reduction of energy and a slowing down of life-giving processes. Co-Enzyme Q10 has been used to help heart problems, high blood pressure, chronic fatigue, gum disease and immune deficiencies.

Alpha lipoic acid

Alpha lipoic acid (ALA) is a powerful antioxidant and its job is to release energy by burning glucose. This, in turn, helps your body store less fat and is so helpful when you are aiming to lose weight. Alpha lipoic acid also support your liver function, which is the waste disposal unit of your body, so helps you to detoxify more efficiently and it plays a role in slowing down the ageing process.

Green tea extract

Green tea (*Camellia sinensis*) is primarily known for its beneficial antioxidants but it also helps with weight loss as it has a fat burning effect.

Siberian ginseng *(Eleutherococcus senticosus).*

Siberian ginseng is a very gentle adaptogenic herb that has a balancing effect on your hormones, in particular the stress hormones. It can provide energy when you need it and can also help you cope when you are under pressure. This makes it less likely that you will find yourself reaching out for comfort food.

Note that Siberian ginseng is a totally different plant from Panax ginseng (also known as Asian, Chinese or Korean ginseng). I would not recommend women take these other kinds of ginseng as they are very strong and can cause palpitations.

This list of vitamins, minerals and other nutrients I believe we could all benefit from taking may seem quite long. That's why I've distilled them all into one good multivitamin and mineral formula, in the right amounts. It's called Nutri Support (see www.naturalhealthpractice.com).

Amino acids

Amino acids are the building blocks of the protein that you eat. There are some amino acids which are especially helpful in helping you to lose weight. These include N-acetyl cysteine, carnitine, tyrosine, arginine, glutamine and branch chain amino acids (leucine, isoleucine and valine).

These amino acids have a variety of benefits including helping to reduce insulin levels, making you more sensitive to insulin, and breaking down fat to release energy. They also help with energy production, appetite suppression, healthy thyroid function, muscle building and the reduction of sugar cravings. In addition, they help your body cope with stress.

It is more convenient to take all these amino acids in one supplement, rather than having to take them separately. The combination I use in my clinic is NHP's Amino Support (see www.naturalhealthpractice.com).

Omega 3 fats

We've talked about the importance of omega 3 essential fatty acids in Chapter 3. Most people, women in particular, along with those have followed no fat and low fat diets, may have become deficient in omega 3s.

Omega 3 fats help your body respond to insulin more effectively, which means that the message to store your food as fat is reduced and more of your food is used as energy. Along with chromium, omega 3 fats can help control your appetite and hunger.

As you eat essential fats, your body makes them more and more complex. The omega 6 fat, linoleic acid (found in nuts, seeds and legumes) is converted to gamma linolenic acid (GLA) found in evening primrose oil. From there these omega 6 fats can be either converted to anti-inflammatory (good) substances or pro-inflammatory (bad) ones. In order for your body to make the conversion into the anti-inflammatory ones, you need good levels of the minerals zinc, magnesium and vitamin B6. This conversion can be blocked by substances such as alcohol and trans fats, high levels of insulin from blood sugar fluctuations, not having enough EPA (see below) and also stress.

Over the years in the clinic I have been testing patients' omega 6 and omega 3 levels and the vast majority of people have too much omega 6 in their blood and not enough omega 3. This can cause inflammation and that manifests as pain, soreness, redness anywhere in the body such as arthritis, inflammatory bowel disorders like ulcerative colitis, skin problems and conditions with 'itis' at the end of the word.

Because of this excess of omega 6, I would suggest that you do not take evening primrose oil, sometimes recommended for premenstrual syndrome, or any omega 6 oils such as starflower or borage, or 3, 6, 9 supplements. If you do have pain or inflammation in your body I would suggest you take the omega 6/3 test to see what your levels are and it can be done with a simple home finger prick sample, see Resources Page 158.

The omega 3 fats; starting with alpha-linolenic acid (ALA) found in flaxseeds, pumpkin, soya and walnuts; are converted into eicosapentaenoic acid (EPA), and docosahexaenoic acid (DHA) which are found naturally in oily fish such as salmon, mackerel and sardines. These produce the anti-inflammatory substances and also help to reduce the pro-inflammatory ones.

So, if you're not a vegetarian or vegan, getting your omega 3s from a fish oil supplement is the most useful for your body as no conversion is needed. Look for one containing 770mg EPA and 510mg DHA per day (I recommend NHP's Omega 3 Support – see www.naturalhealthpractice.com). If you are vegan or vegetarian, look for a supplement containing EPA and DHA which is derived from algae, rather than flaxseed, as it's a more biologically available form. (Unfortunately, it is estimated that only about 10 per cent of the ALA from flaxseeds gets converted – and that is only when circumstances are ideal. If, for example, you are stressed, drinking too much alcohol or not getting enough key nutrients; particularly zinc, magnesium and vitamin B6; then your conversion rate will probably be far less than 10 per cent).

I don't use cod liver oil supplements in my clinic as these are made from extracting the oil from the liver of the fish, which is the most toxic part of the animal. My advice is to use fish oils which are extracted from the body of the fish, so the label will just say fish oil not fish 'liver' oil. (Cod liver oil supplements should not be used when aiming to get pregnant or during pregnancy, as the level of vitamin A is too high. It is OK to use omega 3 fish oil supplements, though, as these can benefit both mother and baby.)

Beneficial bacteria

Your intestines are host to billions of beneficial bacteria. These are vital as they help you manufacture certain nutrients like folate and vitamin K. They also support your immune function, as 70 per cent of your immune system is in your gut. In addition, they help control yeasts like *Candida* and they also improve detoxification.

Research over the last few years has shown that they have another function - helping to control your weight. Scientists have found that gut bacteria are different in overweight people compared to people of normal weight. If they put the gut bacteria from an overweight mouse into a thin mouse (while still eating the same amount of food), the thin mouse will become overweight.

Lactobacillus acidophilus is the main species of beneficial bacteria that colonises the small intestines, whereas *Bifidobacteria* are the main beneficial inhabitants of the large intestines. So you want to take a supplement containing both of these species (with about 22 billion in total). The probiotic I use in my clinic is NHP's Advanced Probiotic Support which is freeze-dried so does not need to refrigerated (useful when travelling) see www.naturalhealthpractice.com.

I would not recommend that you take probiotic drinks as they are often loaded with sugar and also do not have very high levels of the beneficial bacteria.

Your ideal supplement programme

In order to make this supplement programme as practical to follow as possible, I would recommend the following to cover all the above nutrients:

- NHP Nutri Support
- NHP Amino Support
- NHP Omega 3 Support
- NHP Vitamin C Support
- NHP Advanced Probiotic Support

All of these are available from good health food shops or online from www.naturalhealthpractice.com.

In an ideal world, you would follow this supplement protocol for three months, in order to get to your ideal weight. Then you could just switch to a good multivitamin and mineral supplement in place of the Nutri and Amino Support (and keep taking the omega 3, if you won't be eating oily fish, and vitamin C).

If you can only take a couple of supplements, then I would suggest the Nutri Support and Amino Support would be your priority, as they contain the most important nutrients mentioned above.

Further lifestyle tips to help you feel healthier, happier and slimmer

Help with cellulite

This 'orange peel' effect on the skin is notoriously difficult to eliminate. It is found mostly on the thighs and, unfortunately, affects predominantly women because of a difference in cell structure between men and women. The tissue that is affected in cellulite is the subcutaneous tissue just below the surface of the skin. When women's thighs are pinched, we get a pitting and bulging effect but when men's thighs are pinched, their skins folds or furrows instead.

Cellulite is hereditary and can be exacerbated by an accumulation of waste products, smoking, stress and poor lymph flow. It is more common in obesity and during the menopause when connective tissue can become thinner, allowing the fat cells to become bigger. So any measures that help restore connective tissue are going to be helpful.

As you change your way of eating and your body starts to re-balance itself, you will naturally release all those excess toxins and waste products your body was holding onto. Make sure to add in more lecithin-rich foods (eggs, peanuts, apples and cruciferous vegetables) as this nutrient helps to prevent fat deposits from coming to the surface of your skin.

There are some other strategies that can help prevent and improve the appearance of cellulite. Let's take a look:

Body brushing

Daily body brushing is a gentle yet powerful way to encourage lymphatic drainage and the removal of toxins from your body. In so doing, it helps to improve the appearance of cellulite in areas such as the thighs and buttocks, where fats and waste materials tend to accumulate.

Use a natural-fibre brush and always body brush on dry skin. Start at the tips of your shoulders and cover your whole body (except your head) with long, smooth strokes, always brushing towards your heart. At first brush gently as your skin will need to get used to the sensation. It will also go slightly red as you start to increase the circulation in areas which may have become stagnated. Try to do this daily.

Exercise

Exercise can also help reduce cellulite as it helps restore a slim subcutaneous fat layer. As you lose weight, the cellulite will also reduce but it is important that you do not lose weight too rapidly as this can make the appearance of the cellulite worse.

Massage

Using a massage oil for cellulite can be helpful. Oils such as fennel, juniper and grapefruit can work well.

Fennel helps to remove water, as it has diuretic properties, and can also break up the fatty deposits under the skin which are characteristic of cellulite. Juniper helps your body to detoxify and grapefruit helps your body to remove toxins.

Always dilute essential oils in a carrier oil (such as sweet almond, wheatgerm, coconut or sesame). Use 15 drops of essential oil (or a combination of oils) per 30ml (6tsp) of carrier oil.

Cellulite massage oil

   5 drops of fennel

   5 drops of juniper

   5 drops of grapefruit

Add to 30ml of a carrier oil. Massage into affected areas morning and evening.

Help for a sluggish metabolism

We've already looked at the problems of an underactive thyroid in Chapter 5. However, if your thyroid blood test is fine but your basal body temperature is low then it is possible that your metabolism is sluggish.

Your thyroid gland is like a thermostat which regulates your body temperature by secreting two hormones which control how quickly your body burns calories and uses energy.

The thyroid hormones are made from iodine and the amino acid tyrosine. Naturally rich sources of iodine are seafood (especially saltwater fish, such as salmon, sardine, anchovies) and seaweeds such as kelp. Tyrosine is found in foods including almonds, avocados, bananas, pumpkin and sesame seeds.

Help for depression

If you tend to eat when you are depressed and find it hard to break this vicious circle, then it is worth trying to alleviate the depression naturally. Make sure that your blood sugar is under control and that can stop the roller coaster of highs and lows in terms of your mood. There are also a number of natural remedies that can be helpful.

St John's wort *(Hypericum perforatum)*

St John's wort is a common, green plant with yellow flowers that is actually classed as a weed. It grows throughout Europe, Asia and the US and has been used for centuries as a mood booster. The small red dots on its petals contain hypericin, a compound that scientists believe is one of the active ingredients responsible for helping depression.

St John's wort has been very well researched and a large-scale meta-analysis of 29 studies, involving more than 5,000 patients with depression, compared the effects of St John's wort with placebo and standard antidepressants. It found that St John's wort was as effective as standard antidepressants and had fewer side effects[76].

It is thought to work as an antidepressant because it can inhibit the reuptake of serotonin (a brain messenger or neurotransmitter) which is how many of the antidepressant medications work.

One study compared the effects of St John's wort against the antidepressant imipramine The results showed that the St John's wort was 'therapeutically equivalent' to imipramine – in other words, it worked as well as the antidepressant but, interestingly, was better tolerated[77].

St. John's wort has been shown to produce improvements in a number of psychological symptoms including depression, anxiety, apathy, sleep disturbances, insomnia and feelings of worthlessness.

St John's wort interacts with a number of medications so speak to your doctor before taking it.

Vitamin D

You may be depressed because you are deficient in vitamin D. Vitamin D is thought of as the 'sunshine vitamin' and in the winter many people suffer from SAD; seasonal affective disorder. Vitamin D receptors are present in the central nervous system and vitamin D can affect neurotransmitters that are linked to depression.

Research has shown that people with depression have lower levels of vitamin D[78]. Supplementing with vitamin D compared to a placebo showed significant improvement in scores of depression in another study[79]. Public Health England advises everyone to take 400ius of vitamin D from October to April each year.

Food sources of vitamin D are relatively few. It is found in oily fish and eggs (a 100g of grilled salmon contains 284ius of vitamin D and a 100g of tinned pilchards contains 560ius, the yolk of one egg contains about 20ius). Other sources include fortified foods such as margarines and breakfast cereals.

Those most at risk of vitamin D deficiency are those who do not go out much in the daytime, those who do not expose their skin to the sunlight and women who constantly wear make-up or cosmetics with in-built sun protection factors. The tone of your skin affects vitamin D production, so the darker your skin the less your body produces vitamin D. Covering up large areas of skin for religious reasons also reduces vitamin D production. It is estimated that we need about 30 minutes' exposure to the sun every day to produce enough vitamin D to keep us healthy – but it has to be the right kind of sun.

Your body produces the best levels of vitamin D when you are exposed to sunlight within a specific UVB spectrum. In certain parts of the UK; such as northern England, Northern Ireland and Scotland; the sunlight is in the wrong spectrum for most of the year.

The symptoms of a vitamin D deficiency are very subtle (bone pain, muscle weakness) and you may not suspect that lack of vitamin D is affecting your moods. The only way to know for sure is to have a blood test (a home finger-prick test is available, see Resources Page 158). Supplement with the vitamin if needed, and then retest about three months later to make sure your level is within the optimal range.

A question a lot of people ask me, when I give talks, is how much vitamin D should they take? The answer, of course, is that it depends on the level of your deficiency. For this reason, I now recommend that everyone gets their vitamin D level checked, given this nutrient's far-reaching health benefits, and then supplements to get the level back to normal.

There is, though, such a thing as too much vitamin D. A vitamin D level that is too low (less than 10 nmol/L) increases the risk of all-cause mortality (dying of any cause) – but the same is true if your vitamin D level is too high (more than 140 nmol/L)[80]. Similarly, a level of vitamin D that is too low or too high increases an allergic response, such as the response you'd have during a peanut or shellfish allergy[81].

We have known for many years that vitamin D is important for bone health and in the prevention of osteoporosis. However, it is only in recent years that we have realised how important this nutrient is for general health and, particularly, for brain health. Here are just some of the main benefits of vitamin D:

- It in plays a major role in breast and bowel cancer prevention.
- It is important for your immune function, particularly when you need to fight off colds and flu.
- It helps protect your body against conditions as diverse as type 2 diabetes, heart disease, joint pains and arthritis, dementia, infertility, autism and allergies.
- It reduces the risk of SAD (seasonal affective disorder).

Vitamin D balances your immune function (if you have an autoimmune problem it's especially important to have your vitamin D levels tested) as well as helping with depression. And with all the benefits mentioned above, getting your level just right is crucial.

Omega 3

We've all heard of fish being great 'brain food' and there is a reason for this. Your brain is 70 per cent fat, but it needs to the right type of fat. Omega 3 fatty acids are needed for your brain cells to 'pick up' your neurotransmitters so they can be utilised by the brain cells efficiently. So increasing Omega 3 levels can have a direct effect on serotonin.

Previous research has shown a link between depression and low levels of omega 3 fatty acids in blood tests[82]. And now a large analysis of 28 studies has confirmed that EPA is more effective than DHA in treating depression[83].

That is why the amount of EPA in the omega 3 fish oil you are taking is so important. If you are taking a supplement, aim for a level around 770mg EPA and 500mg DHA per day, not just the amount of fish oil mentioned on the front of the supplement. The same if you are taking a vegan EPA/DHA supplement. And if you are concerned about your moods and think they drive you to eat unhealthily, it would be worth finding out if you have enough omega 3 in your body. There is a simple home finger-prick test at www.naturalhealthpractice.com.

Tryptophan

Tryptophan is an important amino acid for mood and depression. Your body makes serotonin from tryptophan. Tryptophan occurs naturally in foods such as dairy products, fish, bananas, dried dates, soya, almonds and peanuts. It's one of the amino acids that is considered essential because our bodies can't manufacture it. Tryptophan is converted into serotonin, unlike conventional antidepressants, which don't 'supply' serotonin but act as selective serotonin reuptake inhibitors (SSRIs), keeping levels of serotonin high in the brain.

Protein is made up of long chains of amino acids. When you eat protein, your body breaks it down into its different amino acids, which then travel into your bloodstream to reach your brain. You have a blood-brain barrier, which controls what gets into your brain, so a competition starts to take place. There are fewer tryptophan molecules than the other amino acids. Therefore, other amino acids get across the barrier leaving the tryptophan behind.

But, if a meal contains a carbohydrate as well, the situation is very different. Carbohydrates help the body to release insulin and the insulin makes use of the other amino acids, leaving the tryptophan to dominate. So combining both protein and carbohydrates together in one meal can be beneficial for mood.

Research has shown that depressed patients have decreased tryptophan levels and a review of a number of studies showed that 5-HTP (5-hydroxytryptophan, a supplement form of tryptophan) was significantly better than a placebo at alleviating depression[84].

B vitamins

The B vitamins, particularly B6, are essential for depression. B6 is involved with the production of neurotransmitters which control mood and behaviour. It's required as a co-enzyme in the production of serotonin. Many antidepressants are formulated to keep serotonin in the brain for longer so, if we have more of this brain chemical to start with, we have more chance of a better mental state.

Also, low levels of both serum folate (a B vitamin) and B12 are associated with a greater risk of depression[85].

It's always best to take a supplement containing a combination of the B vitamins as they all work synergistically, thus when taken together work more effectively.

Aromatherapy essential oils

Aromatherapy oils can also be very useful in lifting your mood. Both bergamot and neroli oils can be added to a bath or used in a massage oil. Ylang ylang and jasmine also have a powerful euphoric effect. As stated before, always dilute essential oils in a carrier oil. Add a total of 15 drops of essential oils to 30ml of a carrier oil, such as sweet almond oil, and shake to blend.

The oils mentioned here are safe for everyone but other essential oils can be contraindicated in pregnancy and with some medical conditions. Always consult a professional aromatherapist if you have a medical condition, are pregnant or breast-feeding.

Exercise

Exercise is important for improving mood. It releases brain chemicals called endorphins, which help us to feel happier, more alert and calmer. These endorphins can have a dramatic and positive effect on the depression, stress and anxiety associated with PMS.

Help for stress

If you eat when you are stressed, then you need to learn to stay calm. Try to keep detached from the problem and take a step back from the stress. You will already have learned about the importance of maintaining your blood sugar levels by eating every three hours. We have also looked at how exercise can be very powerful in helping the management of stress. You can also use mindfulness to help both with stress and depression. Mindfulness-based cognitive therapy has been endorsed by NICE (National Institute for Health and Clinical Excellence) and the National Institutes of Health in the US. It has been shown to help with improving wellbeing and levels of happiness and is as effective as drugs for treating depression[86]. There are many good books, websites and apps that can give you an introduction and practical guide to mindfulness and meditation.

There are also some natural remedies which can help you deal with stress.

Magnesium

Magnesium has a tranquillising, calming effect on your body. It can be combined with the B vitamins, which are well known for their ability to help with stress – try both in supplement form.

Herbs

Herbs really come into their own when it comes to controlling stress. They act on the nervous system to relieve anxiety, tension and irritability, and one of the most well-known is valerian. Valerian is a powerful relaxant and particularly useful if you find that stress is causing insomnia. It can be combined with skullcap which also relaxes the nervous system. Siberian ginseng and rhodiola are both adaptogenic herbs that are also excellent for helping your body and mind when you are stressed.

Aromatherapy oils

Neroli, rose or sandalwood can help calm and relax you. If you are feeling irritable then chamomile, lavender and ylang ylang are good as they can sooth anger, as well as balancing your feelings. Use them in the bath, apply a blend to your pulse points, diffuse it in an oil burner or have someone massage you with an oil blend.

Stress massage oil

5 drops of chamomile

5 drops of lavender

5 drops of ylang ylang

Add these 15 drops to 30ml of a carrier oil, such as sweet almond oil, and shake to blend.

Help with water retention

Water retention is a common symptom and many women find it's particularly bad just before their period. You may find it becomes so bad that you have trouble putting rings on your fingers and shoes on your feet. It can also add a kilo or so to your weight. Your first instinct may be to limit the amount you drink but, in fact, you should do exactly the opposite. It's important to drink *more* water and reduce your intake of salt, including hidden salt in convenience foods. If you limit your intake of water your body will think there is a shortage and try to retain the water you have, hence the retention in the first place.

Many women who suffer from water retention turn to diuretics. These will increase the rate at which fluid is lost but they can also flush important minerals out of your body – for example, potassium which is vital in the correct functioning of your heart. Instead, try these natural remedies to help with water retention.

Dandelion

Dandelion is a natural diuretic that allows fluid to be released without you losing vital nutrients at the same time. It contains more vitamins and minerals than any other herb and is one of the best natural sources of potassium. It is the leaves that are useful for water retention, so take the dried herb in capsule form or pick fresh dandelion leaves and eat them raw in salads. You can use dandelion tea or herbal tea blends containing dandelion but, to have the diuretic effect, the tea needs to be made from the leaves of the dandelion plant. Dandelion coffee will be made from the root.

Parsley

Parsley is not only rich in vitamin C, but is a useful diuretic. It can be taken in capsules or eaten raw.

Aromatherapy oils

Certain aromatherapy oils can also be helpful in countering water retention, particularly fennel. Add 10 drops of fennel to a warm bath and relax in it for 15-20 minutes. Then massage your body using 15 drops of fennel in 30ml (six teaspoons) of a carrier oil such as sweet almond oil.

Help your liver

This vital gland (the largest in the body) is part of our digestive system. Among its many tasks are the storage and filtration of blood, the secretion of bile and numerous metabolic functions, including the conversion of sugars into glycogen. It plays a vital part in fat metabolism and in the oxidation of fat to produce energy. It's worrying, therefore, that in many overweight people liver function can be impaired.

Excess food is converted to fat in the liver and then transported around your body to be stored. Your liver also plays a part in thyroid function by converting thyroxine (T4) into the more active form triiodothyronine (T3). When this conversion is insufficient a person may develop an underactive thyroid (hypothyroidism) which we have looked at in Chapter 5. Your liver is also the 'waste disposal' unit of your body. It detoxifies the body by combining harmful substances like chemicals, drugs, alcohol with less harmful substances which are then excreted by the kidneys.

Certain natural remedies can be used to optimise the functioning of the liver and aid its ability to break down and metabolise fats.

Dandelion

Not just useful for water retention, dandelion is an important liver herb. It is a gentle tonic for the liver and helps to increase the secretion of bile, which assists the digestive system (including the digestion of fat). Rather than the leaves though, you'll need to take a dandelion root supplement.

Milk thistle (Silybum marianum)

Milk thistle is another excellent herb for the liver. Silymarin is the collective name for the substances found in milk thistle which have a beneficial effect. They act as antioxidants which can reduce free-radical production and this is thought to have a detoxifying effect. Milk thistle is the most well-researched plant in the treatment of liver disease[87]. The herb can be taken in capsule form.

Artichoke

Globe artichoke is related to the milk thistle plant and it helps to carry toxins from your liver out of your body by stimulating bile flow. Artichoke has been shown to reduce total cholesterol and improve liver enzymes[88]. It has also been helpful for non-alcoholic fatty liver disease which is the most common cause of liver disease in the world[89].

Help with constipation

There can, of course, be medical reasons for this problem but very often constipation is caused purely by unhealthy eating or drinking. Check with your doctor that you are not taking anything like iron in the form of ferrous sulphate that could be causing the constipation. If you are a sufferer, you should first increase the amount of fibre in your eating plan (as outlined in Chapter 3). However, while you are changing your eating patterns you may need some extra help. The aim is to have comfortable, easy bowel movements every day. If you don't, toxins and waste products that should be eliminated through your bowels can be reabsorbed back into bloodstream.

Normal laxatives work by stimulating or increasing the number of bowel movements or by encouraging a softer or bulkier stool. In theory this sounds good but it's easy to become dependent upon them and even natural laxatives like senna can be quite harsh. The more laxatives are used, the less your body has to do for itself and ultimately your bowel can lose its tone and muscle action and cannot function without help. The other problem with laxatives is that they can cause your food to rush out of your body before the vital nutrients have been absorbed. There are simple things you can do to help yourself.

Increase your fluid intake

Aim for six to eight glasses of water a day. This stops your stools becoming dry and hard which makes it difficult for them to pass along your bowel. It's especially important to ensure a good water intake when you're increasing the fibre in your diet. Remember that herbal teas can count as a glass of water.

Exercise

We know that exercise is good for your general health but it also very helpful for constipation as it helps to increase bowel contractions which move the stools along.

Flaxseeds

This tiny seed can be especially helpful for constipation. Soak one tablespoon (15ml) of whole flaxseeds in water for at least 30 minutes and swallow first thing in the morning or last thing at night (you need to experiment to see which time of day works for you). Flaxseeds act as a bulk-forming kind of laxative and are very mild so can even be used in the long term. Psyllium husks can also be used. There is an excellent powder that I use in the clinic called D-Tox which contains flaxseeds, psyllium husks, dandelion, chlorella and probiotics (see www.naturalhealthpractice.com).

• Control your appetite with a sniff! •

The Smell and Taste Treatment and Research Foundation in America has been looking at the effects of smell and taste on our moods and behaviour for a number of years. It is thought that the cravings for certain foods are often more about craving the aroma than the actual taste. Interestingly, 95 per cent of taste comes from smell and only 5 per cent from the sensation in the mouth. When a smell is inhaled into the nasal cavity, it becomes dissolved in mucus in special olfactory receptors. An electrical signal is then triggered which travels along nerve fibres into the brain. We are able to smell around 10,000 different chemicals through 500 to 1,000 receptors.

Try this simple experiment. Close your eyes and pinch your nose, then ask someone to put different foods into your mouth one at a time. See if you can identity what you are eating. You will find this very interesting because it is extremely difficult to tell what you are eating without being able to smell it.

Sniffing fragrances like bananas and peppermint has been shown to help dieters lose 2.27kg (5lb) or 2 per cent of their total body weight in a month because it seems to subdue the urge to snack[90].

Other research has shown that just smelling olive oil before eating helped people consume less calories and helped them to feel more satisfied with what they had just eaten[91].

Sniffing an aroma when you have a craving could be helpful in changing your appetite. Inhaling the scent of the essential oil of grapefruit has been shown to help reduce appetite and body weight in animals[92]. Keep a bottle of grapefruit essential oil handy for when you might be tempted to have too many snacks or have the urge to binge.

Spice up your life

We are now seeing more research coming out on the benefits of different spices that have been used for centuries around the world. And some of them can be helpful in giving you a bit of extra help with weight loss along with the dietary changes you are making. I have included recipes in this book that include some of the following super-healthy spices.

Turmeric

Turmeric is the yellow spice that is often used in curries. Its active ingredient is curcumin which has had a lot of research focused on its anti-inflammatory effects for conditions like arthritis. Research in animal studies has shown that curcumin can actually help with weight loss and it is also thought to stop the re-growth of fat after someone has lost weight[93].

Capsaicin

A substance called capsaicin is found in chilli peppers and it is the compound that gives peppers their heat. It is suggested that these peppers can help speed up your metabolism and burn fat, as well as helping to curb your appetite[94]. It is thought that the capsaicin's heat may help with a process called thermogenesis where your body can convert fat into heat and so burn more fat, which adds to weight loss. I think it is fine to add chilli peppers, cayenne or paprika to your cooking but I would not recommend taking capsaicin in supplement form as it can cause digestive problems such as heartburn.

Ginger

Like turmeric, ginger also acts as an anti-inflammatory and is thought to help with maintaining healthy joints. It may also have the same thermogenic effects as capsaicin, because it has warming effects in your body. Including these thermogenic ingredients in your diet may boost your metabolism by up to 5 per cent, and increase fat burning by up to 16 per cent[95]. Simmering a few slices of ginger root in boiling water makes a ginger root tea that stimulates and aids digestion. Ginger in food has the same effect.

Cumin

Cumin is another spice that is often found in curries. Research showed that using just 1 teaspoon a day of cumin (added to yogurt) for three months helped people lose three more pounds than those in a placebo group. And those taking the cumin each day lost three times as much body fat (nearly 15 per cent) as the group just taking yogurt alone without cumin. Other benefits included a reduction in LDL 'bad' cholesterol[96]. Cumin in supplement form has also been shown to be as effective in decreasing weight as the weight loss drug orlistat – and was *more* effective in decreasing insulin levels than orlistat[97]. Cumin is thought to help with weight loss by increasing metabolic rate.

I like sprinkling cumin powder, grated ginger and lemon juice over steamed carrots for a simple, healthy side dish.

Cardamom

Cardamom is another spice traditionally used in Indian cooking. It has been shown to help with glucose tolerance in rats fed on a high carbohydrate, high fat diet[98] and further research is planned on humans. It also thought to be good for digestion so people would often have cardamom tea after a meal to reduce flatulence and general digestive discomfort.

Chapter 8

Tests to Help
Shift Those Inches

There are a number of tests available that can help determine what may be preventing successful weight loss. Sometimes we have a gut instinct there's something more going on with our health so; while it's still key to keep up your healthy eating, exercise and lifestyle; it's worth investigating further. These tests can give invaluable insight into understanding your body better and working through the problems that may be holding you back. Let's look at each in turn.

Food intolerances

If you have tried the elimination diet in Chapter 5 and successfully pinpointed the foods you are reacting to, you are probably not only feeling better but are also losing weight more easily. Many people, however, find it quite hard (and confusing) when it comes to reintroducing foods. In this case, a food intolerance test could be useful for you.

If you prefer, you can save time and confusion by doing the test straight away without doing the elimination diet. The choice is yours and relies to a large extent on how quickly you want to see results.

Food intolerances can affect people in different ways but generally symptoms include bloating, water retention, aching joints, fatigue, stuffy nose, skin problems, headaches, digestive problems and weight gain. These are not life-threatening but can of course affect the quality of your life on a daily basis.

The easiest way to test for food intolerances is to do a blood test. The test measures IgG antibodies to food particles which have leaked through your gut wall. Instead of your body seeing these particles as food, it views them as foreign substances and sends out IgG antibodies to cope with them.

The results of this test can show you how sensitive you are to up to 220 different foods and drinks including dairy, fruits, vegetables, fish, poultry, meat, nuts, grains, yeast, chocolate, sugar and coffee. The sensitivity is rated from elevated, through borderline to normal.

This is an easy test to do as my clinic organises for the lab to send you a kit and you take a simple finger-prick blood sample at home and then send it back to the lab to be analysed. You would then come in for a consultation to go through the results.

Leaky gut (intestinal permeability)

Tracking down the foods to which you are sensitive is only solving half the problem. Why has the problem developed in the first place? What happens when you reintroduce the offending foods to your diet? The answer lies in the state of your intestines, your gut, and its capacity to process food properly. Food intolerances are often a symptom that all is not well with your gut.

This is very important because if your intestines are not functioning properly, you may not be absorbing nutrients efficiently. This means you can become deficient in vital vitamins and minerals.

Your gut should act as a barrier to prevent toxins and large molecules escaping into your bloodstream. If your gut becomes 'leaky', then food particles can escape through your gut wall and give you IgG antibody reactions to foods.

For the test, you swallow a drink containing a mixture of 11 sizes of molecules. The different sizes of molecules in the drink pass through your gut wall and into the bloodstream with differing levels of ease; these molecules are used as 'marker molecules'. You then provide a urine sample and, when this is analysed, the amount of the marker molecules detected in your urine will give a strong indication of how leaky your gut is.

If the test shows you have a leaky gut, you will be given recommendations as to how to heal it using natural remedies. You can then re-test in three months time to make sure that it is back to normal. See Resources, page 158, for information on how to contact my clinic to organise this test.

Candida antibody test

If you read the *Candida* symptoms in Chapter 5 and felt you may be suffering from some of them, you may benefit from this simple finger-prick blood test, where the sample is collected at home (my clinic sends you out a kit). If you have a *Candida* overgrowth, *Candida* antibodies are picked up in your blood which indicates that your body is trying to fight the yeast infection. You would then be given recommendations as to how to change your diet, what to take to replenish beneficial bacteria and how to eliminate the *Candida* overgrowth.

Genetic testing

As you have seen in Chapter 1 there are so many diets out there – Atkins, Dukan, 5:2, cabbage soup, high fibre, low carbohydrate, paleo – it's easy to get confused. No single diet will work for everybody because we are all so different.

I have given you the tools in this book for long-term weight loss and it really does become a way of life rather than a way of eating. You're not only changing your body shape and your weight, you're also transforming your health.

With genetic science ever advancing, it's now possible to take another step forward in understanding how best to eat for your own personal health and optimum weight. DNA tests are available that identify the best balance of foods and the type of exercise that suits your genes.

Results have shown that if people follow a healthy eating plan based on their genetic results, then they lose 33 per cent more weight than those who are on an untailored plan[99].

Tests like this measures genetic markers, which tell you:

- Your nutrient needs, such as omega 3, vitamin D, folate, antioxidants and the B vitamins.
- How well you detoxify.
- Your salt, alcohol and caffeine sensitivities.
- Whether you have a genetic predisposition to be lactose intolerance.
- Carbohydrate and fat response.
- Your optimal way to eat, for example low carbohydrate, Mediterranean.
- Whether you are at risk of Coeliac disease.
- What type of exercise you should be doing that suits your genetic make-up (cardio or weights).
- Your risk of injury and recovery profile.

Knowing this information is important for your general health because you might need higher levels of certain nutrients, you might need to be careful about gluten or dairy or your body might need extra help detoxifying. It is also important for your future health because what you learn about your genetic make-up can help you work on prevention. Think of it more as an extra insight than a diet in itself.

You can see that tests can be useful in finding out what may causing you to hold onto your weight, so if you would like to obtain any of these tests then do get in touch (my clinic details are on the Resources page 158).

Chapter 9

Putting the Plan into Action

You have already learned which foods to include in your new, healthy, natural weight loss plan (back in Chapter 3). But often it can be hard to stick to healthy eating, particularly if you are feeding your family as well as yourself. The meal plans in this chapter assume that you will probably only be cooking for others once a day and able to choose your own food for breakfast and lunch. If you are at home during the week it makes the choice of food much easier, but many of us are at work during day and our choice is restricted

Most of us do not have much time for preparing meals except when we are expecting guests, so meals on a day-to-day basis need to be quick and easy to prepare and yet healthy and nutritious. Therefore, the recipes I have given for the meal plans are mainly quick and simple – with just a few being more involved, for when you have more time. They can all be adapted to suit how much time you have and what you have available in your store cupboard.

Remember if the foundations of what you eat – during your day-to-day work and home life – are healthy, it's not a disaster if you sometimes include less healthy foods when you eat out (it's that 80:20 rule).

Give the old favourites a healthy boost

Your favourite dishes can often be easily made more natural and healthy (and weight reducing). You can easily substitute wholemeal flour for white flour, organic eggs for battery eggs, soya milk for animal milk, maple syrup for sugar (weight-for-weight the same). Remember that if a food is described as 'sugar-free', this does not mean that it isn't sweet – look out for recipes made from naturally sweet ingredients rather than sugar.

I have included meals for a week with extra recipes for variations. If you are working and have limited choice of food for lunch, you could have sandwiches a couple of days a week and take something slightly more substantial on the others.

Remember, this is just to get you started – not a plan to stick to slavishly. Variety is a hugely important part of healthy eating, so once you've got to grips with choosing healthy, whole-food ingredients, and trying new recipes and tastes, it's over to you to get creative.

Daily menus

Monday

Breakfast: Choose a good sugar-free muesli with nuts and seeds and soak overnight in apple or orange juice or make your own (see Recipes).

Mid-morning snack: Oatcakes with tahini.

Lunch: Small jacket potato with tuna, sweetcorn and salad.

Mid-afternoon snack: Apple with a few Brazil nuts.

Dinner: Rainbow Trout (see Recipes).

Tuesday

Breakfast: Porridge oats – buy organic if possible and cook with water. Top with ground nuts or seeds.

Mid-morning snack: Apple and a few almonds.

Lunch: Homemade Carrot and Cashew Soup (see Recipes) or buy a tinned or fresh soup with good ingredients.

Mid-afternoon snack: Celery with hummus.

Dinner: Baked Cod (see Recipes).

Wednesday

Breakfast: Wholemeal or rye toast plus poached or boiled egg with tomatoes or avocado.

Mid-morning snack: Pear with pumpkin seeds.

Lunch: Smoked mackerel and salad.

Mid-afternoon snack: Bio yogurt and seeds.

Dinner: Vegetable Lasagne (see Recipes).

Thursday

Breakfast: Natural live yogurt or kefir with your choice of fresh fruit.

Mid-morning snack: No-sugar nut bar.

Lunch: Vegetable stir-fry with cashew nuts and wholegrain rice.

Mid-afternoon snack: Guacamole with vegetable crudités.

Dinner: Fish Cakes (see Recipes) served with Tasty Carrots and Parsnips (see Recipes) and salad.

Friday

Breakfast: Slice of wholemeal or wheat-free toast, poached or boiled egg with extra vegetables.

Mid-morning snack: Handful of blueberries and almonds.

Lunch: Your choice of sandwich (see Recipes).

Mid-afternoon snack: Two oatcakes with nut butter.

Dinner: Hazelnut and Courgette Roast (see Recipes) served with salad and sweet potatoes (see Recipes).

Saturday

Breakfast: Natural live yogurt or kefir with fresh fruit salad topped with ground seeds.

Mid-morning snack: No-sugar cereal bar.

Lunch: Tuna and Brown Rice Salad (see Recipes).

Mid-afternoon snack: Apple and a few mixed nuts.

Dinner: Bouillabaisse (see Recipes) served with salad.

Sunday

Breakfast: Poached egg on wholemeal, rye or sourdough toast with grilled tomatoes and mushrooms.

Mid-morning snack: Bio-yogurt with seeds.

Lunch: Grilled Salmon Steaks with Teriyaki Sauce (see Recipes) served with Stir-fry Vegetables and Curried Rice.

Mid-afternoon snack: Apple with almonds.

Dinner: Stir-fry vegetables and noodles.

Conclusion

As I hope you will have realised by now, this way of eating is not a quick-fix solution. I'm not promising that you'll shed half a stone in a week or that you'll drop four dress sizes in a month. But, as I also hope you'll realise, this is exactly why it works – long-term. Follow this plan and you *will* lose weight – slowly, safely, gently, naturally. Anything worthwhile is going to require commitment and effort. When we learn any new skill it takes a few weeks before it becomes second nature and it is exactly the same with learning to eat differently. After a short while, your new eating pattern will be effortless and automatic.

Remember that when you lose weight too quickly you will simply put it right back on the moment you return to your old eating habits. The key to long-term weight loss is, as we've seen, changing your eating patterns and lifestyle. When you do that, just watch the weight come off! Yes, it will be gradual but it will stay off and you will start feeling wonderful, because this plan isn't just about losing weight, it's about taking control of your health and happiness – now and for all your life.

You may have spent years focusing on losing weight. If you make *health* your goal rather than just inch loss, your whole perspective and relationship with food will change. Once that happens, your weight will automatically change, too. As Hippocrates said: 'Let food be thy medicine'.

Over a number of years, scientists have been looking at nutrition in a different light. They have realised that what we eat can have a role in the prevention of a whole host of diseases: heart disease, cancer, osteoporosis, arthritis, type 2 diabetes, as well as premature ageing and many common conditions including acne, high blood pressure, infertility, irritable bowel syndrome and premenstrual syndrome.

Degenerative disease is *not* inevitable. In other cultures, where people eat different foods, in different environments to us, they are often free from our range of health problems. Yet, if those people move to the West or, alternatively, if they adopt our lifestyle and diet into their culture then 'our' illnesses invariably start to appear.

As scientists learn more about the power of food, it is possible that Thomas Edison may be right when he said: 'The doctor of the future will give no medicine but will interest his patient in the care of the human frame, in diet and in the cause and prevention of disease'.

So persevere with making the lifestyle recommendations in this book and see not only your weight change but also your health.

Welcome to a brand new you – and a whole new way of living. Good luck!

Marilyn

Marilyn

The Recipes

For Breakfast

Home-made muesli (per serving)

Use **raw ingredients** of your choice, preferably organic whole grain cereals.

1oz per serving of one of the following: oats, rice flakes, millet flakes, barley flakes, rye flakes or buckwheat flakes.

1 ½ heaped tbsps of whole or freshly ground seeds (flaxseeds, pumpkin, pine kernels and/or sesame)

½ tbsp of whole or crushed fresh nuts (optional) (almonds, Brazils, cashews, pecan and/or hazelnut)

1 good handful of mixed fresh fruit – for example: banana, mango, pear, peach, kiwi or berries.

Serve with ⅓ pint oat milk, rice milk, or organic soy milk. 1 tbsp of goat, sheep or organic live plain yogurt could also be used.

Protein kick start

Blend the following:

1 cup of frozen mixed berries (strawberries, blueberries, raspberries, blackcurrants, blackberries) and ½ banana or other fruit of choice

5 fl oz rice, oat, soy milk or filtered water

5-6 fl oz filtered water

1 heaped tbsp ground almonds and seeds (sesame, pumpkin, flaxseeds, pine kernel) and 1 tbsp flax oil

Breakfast omelettes

Beat together two eggs with 2 tbsp of non-dairy milk. Heat a small tsp of organic olive oil or organic butter in a small frying pan and pour in the egg mixture. Carefully stir the egg to fold the mixture. When nearly set, add a filling of tomato, onions, red pepper.

Millet, quinoa or oat porridge (do not use quick oats)

Made with ⅓ pint of oat, rice or almond milk or water and sprinkled with 2 tbsp ground nut/seed mixture

Grilled sardines, herrings or mackerel fillets

Served on rye toast or other wheat-free option

Berry booster

Blend together a 9oz pot of natural sheep's, plain organic live or soya yogurt with 2 tbsp mixed berries, 1 tbsp ground mixed seeds/nuts and 1 tbsp flax seed oil. N.B. other fruits may be used such as bananas, kiwis, mangoes, peaches, pears, plums

For Lunch

Sandwiches

Choose wholemeal bread, spelt, sourdough or rye. Wholemeal pitta can also make a change from sliced bread.
Suggestions for fillings include:
tahini and freshly sliced apple
hummus and salad
mashed avocado with a sprinkling of sunflower seeds
bean sprouts and tahini
tofu mashed with a little miso and salad
tuna and salad
miso, tahini, lettuce and a squeeze of lemon
egg and cress
avocado and salad

Soups

Fresh Tomato Soup

Serves 4-6

750g (1lb 10oz) firm tomatoes
15ml (1 tbsp) extra virgin olive oil
1 large garlic clove, very finely chopped
A few sprigs of fresh basil, marjoram or parsley
750ml (1¼ pints/3 cups) vegetable stock or water
Salt and freshly ground black pepper (both optional)

Plunge the tomatoes into boiling water for about 15 seconds, then cool in running cold water. Peel and chop the tomatoes roughly, taking care not to lose any of the juice. Heat the oil gently in a saucepan and sauté the tomatoes for a couple of minutes. Add the garlic and herbs and simmer with the lid off the pan for just 5 minutes. Put in the stock or water, salt and pepper, cover the pan and cook for a further 5 minutes only. To ensure a lovely fresh taste, do not overcook. This soup can be served hot, but is even better chilled in summer.

Spicy Carrot and Parsnip Soup

Serves 6

225g (8oz) carrots, chopped
450g (1lb) parsnips
1 onion, chopped
30ml (2 tbsp) olive oil
15ml (1 tbsp) curry powder
350ml (12 fl oz) organic milk or non-dairy alternative
5ml (1 tsp) sea salt
10ml (2 tsp) cumin seeds

If the carrots and parsnips are organic, then there is no need to peel them: just scrub them clean. Cut the parsnips in half and remove the woody centre. Cut both the parsnips and carrots into even-sized pieces.

Heat the oil in a heavy saucepan, add the vegetables and stir to coat with oil. Add the curry powder and stir for 1 minute. Stir in the vegetable stock and milk and season to taste. Bring to the boil and then gently simmer for 20 minutes or until the vegetables are soft.

Blend the mixture in a food processor until smooth. Toast the cumin seeds by gently roasting in a frying pan without oil but stirring constantly. Use the seeds as a garnish.

This soup can also be made with pumpkin or squash instead of carrots and also with any other mixture of root vegetables.

Salads

Tuna Fish Salad

Serves 4

15ml (tbsp) cider vinegar
45ml (3 tbsp) olive oil
5ml (1 tsp) mustard (optional)

Juice of ½ lemon

225g (8oz) cooked organic brown rice or quinoa

200g (7oz) can tuna fish in spring water, drained

A few drops of soya sauce

5cm (2in) cucumber, finely chopped

15ml (1 tbsp) chopped parsley

In a screw top jar, combine the vinegar, oil, mustard (if using) and lemon juice and then shake until mixed thoroughly.

Place the cooked rice (or quinoa) in a large bowl and pour over the oil and vinegar mixture. Flake the tuna and add to the bowl. Add the soya sauce, cucumber and parley and mix thoroughly.

Watercress and Orange Salad

Serves 2

1 large bunch of watercress

2 navel oranges

20ml (2 tbsp) walnut halves, crushed

8-10 olives

For the dressing

Half a garlic clove, crushed

1.5 ml (¼ tsp) sea salt

5ml (1 tsp) wholegrain mustard

Freshly ground black pepper

60ml (4 tbsp) extra virgin olive oil

15ml (1 tbsp) balsamic vinegar

Wash the watercress in several changes of water, then pick over carefully, discarding any slightly yellowed leaves and the thick stems. Dry thoroughly. Slice the oranges, removing any pith and pips, then cut each slice into eight pieces.

To make the dressing, mash the garlic and salt with the back of a spoon to be sure the garlic is well crushed. Combine with the mustard, pepper, oil and vinegar. Just before serving, put the watercress, orange, walnuts and olives in a salad bowl, pour over the dressing and toss.

For Dinner

Rainbow Trout

Serves 4

4 x 175g (6oz) rainbow trout, cleaned
2 medium onions, peeled and chopped
5ml (1 tsp) sea salt
Pinch of freshly ground pepper
250ml (8 fl oz/1 cup) vegetable stock or optional white wine
4 lemon wedges
Sprigs of parsley

Preheat the oven to 180°C (350°F/gas mark 4). After rinsing the trout under cold water, pat them dry and arrange them in a shallow baking dish. Sprinkle with the onions, salt and pepper. Pour the stock (or wine) over the fish.

Bake for 20 minutes basting occasionally or until the fish flakes when tested with a fork.

Serve garnished with lemon wedges and parsley and accompanied with vegetables and/or salad.

Oven-roasted Pumpkin

Serves 4

This can be enjoyed on its own or served with grilled fish and salad. It goes particularly well with the Watercress and Orange Salad.

1kg (2¼ lb) orange pumpkin
30ml (2 tbsp) extra virgin olive oil
25ml (1 rounded tbsp) rosemary leaves (fresh if possible)
Salt and ground pepper

Preheat the oven to 200°C (400°F/gas mark 6). Peel the pumpkin and cut into slices about 2cm (¾in) thick and roughly 8cm (3in) long. Put into a large bowl and drizzle with the olive oil. Toss to coat the pumpkin thoroughly then sprinkle with rosemary, salt and pepper, mixing well.

Spread the pumpkin slices in a baking dish, making sure any rosemary leaves stuck in the bowl are transferred to the pumpkin. Bake for about 20 minutes, until the pumpkin is golden brown underneath, then turn and bake for a further 20 minutes or longer until the pumpkin is very tender and fragrant. Serve hot.

Vegetable Casserole

Serves 4

This recipe can be made in large quantities and kept refrigerated. It's good hot, but equally delicious at room temperature as a salad. You can omit or replace some of the vegetables if you like: pumpkin, giant white radish, parsnip or okra can all be used in this dish.

60ml (4 tbsp) olive oil
1-2 leeks, sliced
2 sweet potatoes, sliced
4 small carrots, cut into strips lengthways
4 medium onions, peeled and thickly sliced
2 courgettes, thickly sliced
2 red or green peppers, deseeded and cut into strips
1 small aubergine, peeled and sliced
4 large tomatoes, thickly sliced
Sal and ground black pepper to taste
For the garlic-herb mix
4 garlic cloves, finely chopped
100ml (4 rounded tbsp) chopped fresh herbs (including parley, dill, coriander, spring onion, celery tops)

Preheat the oven to 180°C (350°F/gas mark 4). Put a film of oil in a deep casserole dish. Combine the garlic and herbs in a small bowl. Layer the vegetables inside the dish and sprinkle each layer with seasoning, oil and garlic-herb mix. Start with a layer of leeks. Followed by sweet potatoes, then the other vegetables finish with a layer of tomatoes so that their moisture will seep down through the rest of the vegetables during cooking. Drizzle over the rest of the oil, cover the dish securely and bake in the oven for 45-60 minutes until the vegetables are tender but not mushy.

Vegetable Lasagne

Serves 4

This is an excellent dish for serving up lentils to those who don't normally eat them. Seaweed is also used in this dish but in such a way that you can't taste it, yet you get all the valuable trace ingredients, so it is a very easy way of introducing it into the diet. You can use the same filling as a vegetarian shepherd's pie and also use sweet potatoes for the topping as a change from ordinary potatoes.

175g (6oz) brown lentils
5cm (2in) piece kombu seaweed

1 medium onion, peeled and sliced
1 garlic clove, crushed
15ml (1 tbsp) extra virgin olive oil
400g (14oz) canned tomatoes
Pinch of mixed dried herbs
5ml (1 tsp) soya sauce or tamari
5ml (1 tsp) miso
15ml (1 tbsp) sugar-free tomato ketchup
1 packet wholewheat or wheat-free lasagne, cooked

In a pressure cooker or heavy saucepan with a lid, put the brown lentils together with the piece of kombu and enough water to cover. Cook until the lentils are soft, adding more water if necessary.

Lightly sauté the sliced onion with the garlic in the olive oil in a large frying pan or wok (you need a pan with slightly higher sides than a regular frying pan) until they are soft. Add the canned tomatoes and mixed herbs.

When the lentils are cooked, drain them, saving any excess cooking water, and add them to the tomato mixture. Keeping the heat low, stir well. Add the soya sauce, miso and ketchup. As you get used to cooking this dish, you can alter these last ingredients to suit your taste. Simmer for 5 minutes more.

Put the lentil mixture in a blender for just a short while with a little of the reserved lentil cooking water. This mixture forms the layers of the dish so it needs to be firm and not too runny.

In a rectangular baking dish, put one layer of pasta, then one layer of sauce and keep layering until the pasta is the top layer. You can add a sprinkling of grated cheese if desired.

Place in a preheated oven at 180°C (350°F/gas mark 4) until the pasta is slightly golden.

Baked Cod

Serves 4

1 medium onion, peeled and sliced
75ml (5 tbsp) extra virgin olive oil
550g (1lb 4oz) thick cod fillet, skinned and cut into pieces
3 large tomatoes, cut into wedges
30ml (2 tbsp) capers
75g (3oz) olives
30ml (2 tbsp) fresh chopped parsley

Preheat the oven to 200°C (400°F/gas mark 6).

Sauté the onion in just 5ml (1 tsp) of the olive oil until cooked and slightly brown.

Put the cod in a large baking tin with the tomatoes. Sprinkle over the onions, capers and olives and drizzle with the rest of the olive oil.

Bake for 20 minutes or until the fish is cooked (it should flake easily).

Sprinkle with the parsley and serve with vegetables or a salad.

Fish Cakes

Makes 12

550g (1lb 4oz) potatoes
225g (8oz) undyed smoked haddock
60ml (4 tbsp) milk or soya milk
15ml (1 tbsp) lemon juice
30ml (2 tbsp) fresh chopped parsley
Sea salt and ground pepper to taste
15ml (1 tbsp) extra virgin olive oil

Boil the potatoes in lightly salted water for 20 minutes. While the potatoes are cooking, rest a plate over the boiling water and poach the fish in the soya milk. It is cooked when the fish is firm. Mash the drained potatoes with the poaching soya milk. Add the flaked fish to the potatoes. Beat in the lemon and parsley and season to taste. Leave the mixture to cool.

Divide the mixture into 12 and shape into cakes about 1cm (½in) thick. Lightly oil a frying pan and fry the fish cakes for 5 minutes on each side.

Tasty Carrots and Parsnips

This recipe is so simple and yet so tasty! The quantities are vague so that you can design this dish to your taste, especially in terms of the garlic and ginger. Enjoy it as a side or a light dish on its own.

Carrots
Parsnips
5 ml (1 tsp) extra virgin olive oil
Fresh root ginger, peeled and grated, to taste
Garlic, crushed, to taste
Tamari or soya sauce, to taste
5ml (1 tsp) maple syrup or to taste

If the carrots and parsnips are organic, then leave the skins on; otherwise peel. Cut into wedges. Heat the oil in a wok and add in the ginger and garlic. Then add the vegetables and stir for a couple of minutes. Add 250ml (8fl oz/1 cup) of water, the soya sauce and maple syrup. Cover and cook for about 10 minutes until almost all the liquid has evaporated.

Squid with Asian Vinaigrette

Serves 2

A refreshing meal of lightly cooked squid and crunchy vegetables with a tangy Asian dressing.

500g (1c lb) squid
100g (4oz) snow peas, blanched and halved
2 stalks celery, thinly sliced
2-3 shallots, or half a mild onion, finely sliced
115g (4oz) sliced water chestnuts
For the dressing
1 garlic clove, very finely minced
30ml (2 tbsp) rice vinegar
15ml (1 tbsp) lemon juice
15ml (1 tbsp) maple syrup
5ml (1 tsp) soya sauce
2.5ml (½ tsp) sesame oil
Chilli powder, to taste

Wash the squid thoroughly, peeling off and discarding the reddish-brown skin. Pull the beaky part out of the centre of the tentacles and discard this but keep the tentacles. Cut the squid tube into pieces roughly 5x2cm (2x¾in). Bring a pan of lightly salted water to the boil and put in the squid pieces and tentacles. Simmer for about 2 minutes, just until the squid turns white and is lightly cooked. Drain.

Combine all the dressing ingredients. Toss the squid with 30ml (2 tbsp) of dressing and refrigerate for 30 minutes.

Put the marinated squid and all the other ingredients into a serving bowl, add the rest of the dressing and toss well. Serve lightly chilled.

Grilled Marinated Salmon Steaks

Serves 4

4 salmon steaks (wild or organic not farmed), approx. 2.5cm (1in) thick

For the marinade

15ml (1 tbsp) per portion of fish, made up of equal parts of soya sauce, freshly grated ginger and freshly squeezed lemon juice.

Pour the marinade over the salmon and let stand for 5 minutes. Turn the fish over and leave for another 5 minutes. Remove from the marinade and grill for about 3-5 minutes on one side. Turn the fish over, brush with the marinade and grill for another 3-5 minutes. Herbs such as sage or basil can also be sprinkled on top before grilling.

Grilled Plaice with Tomato and Orange Sauce

Serves 4

4 plaice fillets
30ml (2 tbsp) wholemeal flour
15-30ml (1-2 tbsp) olive oil
For the sauce
1 orange
350g (12oz) tomatoes, chopped
2 shallots, finely chopped
1 garlic clove, crushed
15ml (1 tbsp) pure fruit marmalade no added sugar

Coat each fillet with flour and drizzle about 1.5ml (¼ tsp) of oil on the plaice. Grill for about 5 minutes until the fish is cooked.

To make the sauce, grate the orange rind and squeeze the juice. Put 30ml (2 tbsp) of the juice into a pan and stir in the tomatoes, shallots and garlic. Cook over a medium heat for a few minutes. Stir in the marmalade and, after bringing to the boil, simmer for about 20 minutes.

Scrambled Tofu with Sweetcorn

Serves 4

5ml (1 tsp) olive oil
225g (8oz) sweetcorn, frozen is fine
225g (8oz) tofu, plain or smoked
10ml (2 tsp) soya sauce or tamari

Place the olive oil in a pan, then add the sweetcorn and the tofu crumbled into tiny pieces. Warm through by stir frying and add the soya sauce to taste.

Arame seaweed can be added to this recipe: soak 60ml (4 tbsp) in boiling water for 10 minutes or until soft, strain the water. Add the arame to the scrambled tofu and mix well.

Tofu Burgers

Serves 4

225g (8oz) tofu
1 celery stalk, very finely chopped
½ onion, peeled and very finely chopped
½ carrot, grated
Pinch of sea salt
50-75g (2-3oz) wholewheat flour
15ml (1 tbsp) olive oil for each batch of frying

Drain the tofu and pat dry to remove excess moisture. Mash the tofu and mix with the other ingredients, except the oil. Use more or less flour to get the burgers to hold together easily. Heat the oil and fry two or three burgers at the same time for approximately 5 minutes on each side.

For Dessert

Melon Granita

Serves 4

2kg (4½ lb) ripe melons (any melon is fine except watermelon)
Maple syrup if desired

Before you begin, turn the setting on your freezer to maximum. Peel the melons and cut the flesh into chunks. Process a little at a time in a food processor to liquidise the flesh. Put into a bowl and taste for sweetness; if your melon wasn't fully ripe, you may want to add a touch of maple syrup (remembering that chilling food diminishes the sweetness).

Carefully pour the mixture into ice cube trays and freeze for around 5 hours until really firmly set. If you have several very small bowls, you may like to put the additional melon pulp in these in the freezer rather than wait until the first batch in the ice cube trays is ready. If doing the freezing in stages, store each frozen batch in a plastic bag or covered container in the freezer while the next batch chills.

Process the deep frozen melon, just a cupful of cubes at a time, in the food processor until they turn into a slush. Quickly put into a covered container and store in the freezer while doing the next batch of frozen melon cubes. When the whole lot has been processed, it can be stored for several hours or even overnight in the freezer. Take the contain our of the freezer about 15 minutes before serving; if the weather is very hot, you may prefer to leave it in the lower part of the refrigerator rather than on the kitchen work surface before serving. Spoon a little of the melon ice into glass bowls to serve.

Aduki Bean Dessert

Serves 4

225g (8oz) aduki beans
600ml (1 pint/2½ cups) soya milk or other non-dairy milk
Maple syrup
Sliced banana (optional)

Rinse the beans well and, if you've planned in advance, leave them to soak overnight. Otherwise, put them into a saucepan with 600ml (1 pint/2½ cups) of cold water, cover and bring to the boil. Simmer for 10 minutes, then let the beans stand with the pan still covered for up to 1 hour.

Drain the soaked beans well and put into a clean pan with the soya milk. Bring slowly to the boil, stirring, then lower the heat and simmer with lid partially on the pan for 30 minutes. Taste the liquid and add maple syrup to taste. Continue cooking until the beans are really soft and the liquid much reduced, adding a little water if necessary. The amount of time the beans will take to simmer depends on how long you have soaked them initially.

When the beans are soft, serve in small bowls, either hot or at room temperature. The beans can be refrigerated for 2-3 days, but be sure not to serve chilled or the flavour and texture will be spoiled. Top with sliced banana if you wish.

Cracked Wheat Dessert

Serves 4

This recipe could also be made with quinoa, if you want to avoid wheat.

350ml (12 fl oz/1½ cups) bulgur wheat
550ml (18 fl oz/2¼ cups) hot water
6-8 dried apricots, chopped
30-45ml (2-3 tbsp) raisins
120ml (4 fl oz/½ cup) orange juice
120ml (4 fl oz/½ cup) walnut halves, roughly chopped
30-45 ml (2-3 tbsp) pine nuts, toasted in a dry pan until golden
Maple syrup to taste

Put the bulgur in a bowl and pour over the hot water, mixing thoroughly. Leave aside until all the liquid is absorbed and the grains have swollen. Fluff up the mixture with a fork.

While the bulgur is soaking, combine the apricots and raisins with the orange juice and leave them until swollen.

Mix the bulgur, dried fruit and nuts then drizzle in maple syrup to taste. Serve at room temperature. You can serve this with some plain yogurt if you wish.

Baked Bananas

The essence of simplicity, this dessert of grilled bananas is full of flavour and natural sweetness.

1-2 firm ripe bananas per person
5ml (1 tsp) sesame seeds per person
A little ground cinnamon

Put the bananas, still in their skins, under a hot grill and cook, turning frequently, until they are really soft when pierced with a skewer. This should take 10-15 minutes.

While the bananas are cooking, lightly toast the sesame seeds in a dry pan, shaking frequently, until they are golden brown. Turn into a small bowl, sprinkle with cinnamon and set aside.

Just before serving, peel the bananas and lay on a serving dish. Sprinkle over the sesame seeds and cinnamon mixture.

Lemon and Coconut Pancakes

115g (4oz) wholewheat, barley or rye flour
2 organic eggs, beaten
200ml (7fl oz/¾ cup) soya milk or other non-dairy milk
30ml (2 tbsp) olive oil
Juice of 2 lemons
Coconut milk
15ml (1 tbsp) desiccated coconut

Sift the flour into a bowl, make a well in the middle and gradually beat in the eggs, soya milk and oil, either by hand or with a mixer. When smooth, leave to stand for 30 minutes. Heat a small frying pan and brush with oil. Drop 30ml (2 tbsp) of the batter, swill around and cook until bubbles rise and the underside is golden brown. Toss the pancake over and cook the other side.

Put the lemon juice in a mixer with the coconut milk and desiccated coconut and blend. Roll up each pancake with a little sauce in the middle and pour some more sauce over the top of the pancake.

Poached Pears with Carob Custard

Serves 2

2 large pears
45ml (3 tbsp) water
80ml (4 rounded tbsp) rice flour
30ml (2 tbsp) carob flour
750ml (1¼ pints/3 cups) soya or other non-dairy milk
Desiccated coconut, toasted to garnish

Peel, core and quarter the pears and simmer gently in the water until just cooked. Mix the rice flour and the carob flour with a little cold soya milk in a pan until smooth. Add the remaining milk and bring to the boil, stirring all the time. Simmer for 1 minute. Serve the pears with the carob custard and sprinkle with the coconut.

For a special treat, the custard can be made with cacao and a little maple syrup.

Apple Cakes

Makes 16 small cakes

450g (1lb) eating apples
225g (8oz) spelt flour or other flour
10ml (2 tsp) cream of tartar
6ml (1 tsp) baking soda
Pinch of sea salt
115g (4oz) butter
115g (4oz) maple syrup
1 egg

Preheat the oven to 200°C (400°F/gas mark 6) and grease a tray of patty tins. Cook the apples to a puree. Sift together the flour, cream of tartar, baking soda and salt. Cut the butter into small pieces and rub this into the flour until the mixture resembles fine breadcrumbs. Stir in the maple syrup and mix in the beaten egg to form a soft but manageable dough. Knead lightly on a floured surface and roll out 3mm (¹/₈in) thick. Cut out 16 bases and 16 lids.

Line each patty tin with a base, put in a spoonful of the apple puree and put a lid on top. Bake for about 15 minutes.

Bakewell Tarts

These can be made as individual tarts or one big one.

Pastry (can be spelt or other flours)
<u>For the filling</u>
30ml (2 tbsp) pure fruit strawberry jam
50g (2oz) butter
50g (2oz) maple syrup
1 egg, beaten
25g (1oz) ground almonds
1oz wholemeal self-raising flour
A few drops of almond essence
A few drops of vanilla essence

Preheat the oven to 180°C (350°F/gas mark 4). Line a baking dish or small individual tart tins with the pastry. Spread a layer of jam on top of the pastry. Blend all the other ingredients together and add on top of the jam. Bake until lightly brown and a knife when inserted comes out clean.

Baked Apples with Sultanas

4 eating apples
4 tbsp organic sultanas (no minerals or preservatives)
4 tsp water
½ tsp cinnamon

Preheat the oven to 190°C or gas mark 5.

Core the apples and put in a greased small ovenproof dish. In a bowl, mix the sultanas with the water and cinnamon and put 1 tbsp of the mixture in the holes in the apples. Bake in the oven for 40 mins or until soft. Serve with goat, sheep, soya or plain live yogurt.

Rice Pudding

100g easy-cook brown rice
1 cup of raisins (without mineral oil and preservative)
600ml (1 pint) unsweetened soy milk, rice milk, oat milk
1 tsp allspice
1 tsp cinnamon

Grease an oven proof dish. Wash the rice and sprinkle it into the base of the dish. Add the raisins and milk and sprinkle the cinnamon and allspice evenly over the surface. Cover, preferably with a glass lid then bake in the oven for 2 hours.

Banana and Custard

For the custard

2 large egg yolks

1 heaped tsp cornflour or arrowroot

1 tsp of vanilla extract or 1 fresh vanilla pod

300ml (10 fl oz) unsweetened soy, rice, oat milk

In a heatproof bowl, beat the egg yolks, cornflour or arrowroot and vanilla extract (or scrape the inside of the vanilla pod). Warm the milk and pour into the egg mixture. Mix together and return to the pan and stir over a low heat until the mixture coats the back of the spoon or reaches your desired consistency.

Slice up the desired number of bananas into a bowl and pour over the custard.

Buckwheat pancake with fruit and yogurt

1 cup buckwheat flour

2 organic eggs, beaten

1 cup of soya milk or other dairy alternative

A pinch of salt

A small amount of olive oil

In a bowl mix the flour and eggs and slowly add the milk. Stir well to remove any lumps. Add the pinch of salt.

Heat the frying pan and add a small amount of olive oil. Once heated add enough mixture to coat the frying pan. Cook the pancakes both sides.

Serve with fresh fruit compote and organic plain non-dairy yogurt. Sprinkle with chopped nuts or seeds.

Fruity semolina

Semolina is made from wheat so should be avoided if you have an allergy or intolerance to wheat.

150 ml (5 fl oz) soymilk or other milk alternative

2 heaped tsps semolina

1 cup of mixed berries (add a little less fluid if you use frozen fruit)

Put the milk into a saucepan and add the semolina. Heat gently, stirring all the time, for 5 mins or until the liquid thickens. Blend the berries and pour into the semolina. Serve hot or cold.

Mixed berry fool

450g (1lb) mixed berries (frozen or fresh)
225g (8oz) soft tofu, chilled
Dash of vanilla extract
Soya milk, as required

Reserve a few berries for decoration. Put all the ingredients, except the soya milk, in a blender and process well until smooth. Add the soya milk to achieve the required thickness (it should be like cream whipped to soft peaks). Spoon the mixture into clear glasses and decorate with the berries. Chill before serving.

Resources

Glenville Nutrition Clinics

Natural Healthcare For Women

Consultations:

If you would like to have a consultation (either in person, on the telephone or by Skype), then please feel free to phone my clinic for an appointment.

All the qualified nutritionists who work in my UK and Irish clinics have been trained by me in my specific approach to nutrition.

The clinics are located in:

UK - Harley Street, London and Tunbridge Wells, Kent.

For more information or to book a personal or telephone appointment in the UK, please contact us at:

Tel: 01892 515905 | Int. Tel: + 44 1 892 515905
Email: health@marilynglenville.com
Website: www.marilynglenville.com

Ireland - Dublin, Galway and Kilkenny

For more information or to book a personal or telephone appointment in Ireland, please contact us at:

Tel: 01 402 0777 | Int. Tel: + 353 1 402 0777
Website: www.glenvillenutrition.ie

Dubai - The Retreat, Palm Dubai

For more information or to book a personal or telephone appointment in Dubai, please contact us at:

Tel: 04 524 777 | Int. Tel: + 353 1 402 0777
Int. Tel: + 971 4 524 7712
Email: info@gncuae.com
Website: www.rayyawellness.com/glenville-nutrition-clinic

Workshops and Talks: I frequently give workshops and talks. See my website for my upcoming schedule: www.marilynglenville.com. If you would like to organise a workshop/talk near you, I would be happy to come and speak - call my clinic and ask for information about how to arrange this.

Supplements and Tests: The Natural Health Practice (NHP) is my supplier of choice for all the supplements and tests mentioned in this book. They only carry products that I use in my clinics and are in the correct form, the right levels and use the highest quality ingredients. For more information, please contact:

Website: www.naturalhealthpractice.com
Tel: 01892 507598 **Int Tel:** +44 1 892 507598

Online Programme

If you feel that you would like support in losing weight, taking control of your eating pattern, getting your health back and learning about an enjoyable way of eating that becomes a way of life, then join me on my online programme. This programme is not only about how you look and feel now but also your health for the rest of your life. It's also about getting rid of tiredness, not sleeping well, mood swings, irritability, anxiety, food cravings and getting back the quality of life you deserve. For more information or to book your place email health@marilynglenville.com

If you have enjoyed this book then please send a review.
I also invite you to join me on Facebook and Twitter for more information, tips and updates on my work.

/DrGlenvillePhD   @DrGlenville

Free Health Tips

If you would like to receive my exclusive Heath Tips by email, drop me a line at health@marilynglenville.com. Just mention 'Free Health Tips' in the subject line and you will be added to my special list to receive regular health tips and other useful information.

Other Books by Dr Marilyn Glenville PhD

Natural Solutions for Dementia and Alzheimer's

Natural Alternatives to Sugar

Fat Around The Middle - And How To Get Rid Of It

Natural Solutions To The Menopause

Osteoporosis - How To Prevent, Treat And Reverse It

Healthy Eating For The Menopause

Natural Solutions To PCOS

Natural Solutions To IBS

Getting Pregnant Faster

Overcoming PMS The Natural Way

The Natural Health Bible For Women

The Nutritional Health Handbook For Women

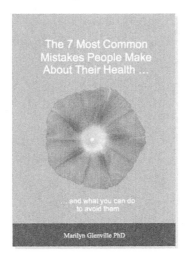

worth £7.77

FREE eBook

The 7 Most Common Mistakes You Are Probably Making About Your Health

And What You Can Do To Avoid Them.

by Dr Marilyn Glenville PhD

Download Here
www.marilynglenville.com/7mistakes

And receive FREE daily natural health tips and advance notification of Dr Glenville's public speaking events

Other books by Dr Marilyn Glenville PhD

Natural Solutions For Dementia And Alzheimer's

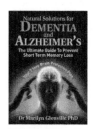

Find out how you can eliminate and prevent short term memory loss, forgetfulness and increase your brain power.

Natural Alternatives To Sugar

It's time to ditch the sugar, banish those sugar cravings once and for all and enjoy a healthy sugar-free life – and this book will show you how.

Fat Around The Middle

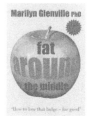

A practical action plan showing how you can get rid of that bulge once and for all…. and it's not just about diet!

Natural Solutions To Menopause

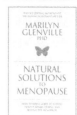

At last the definitive guide to a drug-free, symptom-free menopause and enjoying a long and healthy life beyond it.

Osteoporosis - How To Prevent, Treat And Reverse It.

This ground-breaking book offers you help and advice that combines natural alternatives with conventional treatments.

Healthy Eating For The Menopause

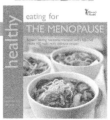

Over 100 great recipes that are tasty enough for the whole family to enjoy and designed to help eliminate your menopause symptoms and keep you healthy.

Getting Pregnant Faster

Boost your fertility in just 3 months and discover the "8 steps to fertility" plan that will help you to get pregnant faster.

Natural Solutions To PCOS

Beat PCOS and enjoy a symptom-free life, naturally. Dr Marilyn Glenville PhD has helped thousands of women overcome PCOS and now you too can benefit from her unique, nutritional programme.

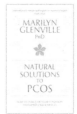

Natural Solutions To IBS

How to relieve the symptoms of IBS and heal your digestive system. Full of practical nutritional advice, as well as suggestions for ways to help tackle emotional wellbeing, this brilliant book offers·the vital support you need.

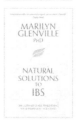

Overcoming PMS The Natural Way

Are you one of the 70% to 90% of women who suffer every month with premenstrual symptoms? At last a groundbreaking approach to eliminating these symptoms for good.

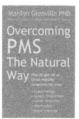

The Natural Health Bible For Women

A practical, easy-to-use reference book guiding you step-by-step through the unique aspects of a woman's body. You will learn how nutrition, lifestyle and natural therapies can maximise your health and vitality.

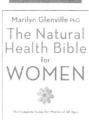

Nutritional Health Handbook For Women

Everything you need to know on the most effective ways to treat all aspects of women's health - naturally.

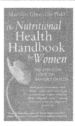

Order directly from: www.naturalhealthpractice.com
or call 01892 507598 and place your order now.

References

[1] https://www.independent.co.uk/voices/comment/52-is-just-the-latest-britain-s-diet-industry-is-worth-2-billion-so-why-do-we-buy-into-it-8737918.html

[2] http://news.bbc.co.uk/1/hi/business/2725943.stm

[3] https://www.nhs.uk/news/obesity/half-of-uk-obese-by-2030/#what-were-the-main-findings

[4] https://www.ncbi.nlm.nih.gov/pmc/articles/PMC2672390/

[5] Jeffrey, RW et al, 1996, Does Weight Cycling Present a Health Risk? Amer J Clin Nutr, 1996, 63 (3 Suppl), 452S-5S

[6] Kim MK et al, 2018, Associations of variability in blood pressure, glucose and cholesterol concentrations and body mass index with mortality and cardiovascular outcomes in the general population, Circulation, 1 Oct.

[7] Cornelissen PL et al, 2009, Patterns of subcutaneous fat deposition and the relationship between body mass index and waist-to-hip ratio: implications for models of physical attractiveness, J Theor Bio, 256, 3, 343-50

[8] De Laet et al , 2005, Body Mass Index as a predictor of fracture risk: A meta-analysis, Osteo Int, 16, 1330-38.

[9] Allaz AF et al, 1998, Body weight preoccupation in middle age and ageing women: a general population survey, Int J Eat Disord, 23, 3, 287-94.

[10] Golay A et al, 2000, Similar weight loss with low-energy food combining or blanced diets, Intern J Obes, 24, 492-496

[11] Tobias DK et al, 2015, Effect of low fat diet interventions versus other diet interventions on long term weight change in adults: a systematic review and meta-analysis, Lancet Diabetes and Endocrinology, 3, 12, 968-979

[12] Hall KD et al, 2016, Energy expenditure and body composition changes after an isocaloric ketogenic diet in overweight and obese men, Am J Clin Nutr, 104, 2, 324-33

[13] Seidelmann SB et al, 2018, Dietary carbohydrate intake and mortality: a prospective cohort study and meta-analysis, Lancet Public Health, August 16, doi: 10.1016/S2468-2667(18)30135-X

[14] Kosinski C and Jornayvax FR, 2017, Effects of ketogenic diets on cardiovascular risk factors: evidence from animal and human studies, Nutrients, 9, 5, 517

[15] Trepanowski JF et al, 2017, Effect of Alternate-Day Fasting on Weight Loss, Weight Maintenance, and Cardioprotection Among Metabolically Healthy Obese Adults A Randomized Clinical Trial, *JAMA Intern Med.* 2017;177(7):930-938

[16] Gabel K et al, 2018, Effects of 8 hour time restricted feeding on body weight and metabolic disease risk factors in obese adults. A pilot study, Nutr Healthy Aging, 4, 4, 345-353.

[17] https://www.nationalgeographic.com/foodfeatures/evolution-of-diet/

[18] http://www.fao.org/docrep/007/y5609e/y5609e02.htm

[19] Samraj AN et al, 2015, A red meat-derived glycan promotes inflammation and cancer progression, Proc Natl Acad Sci USA, 112, 2, 542-547

[20] https://www.nationalgeographic.com/foodfeatures/evolution-of-diet/

[21] Osterdahl M et al, 2008, Effects of a short-term intervention with a paleolithic diet in healthy volunteers, Eur J Clin Nutr, 62, 5, 682-5

[22] Huang R et al, 2016, Vegetarian Diets and Weight Reduction: a Meta-Analysis of Randomized Controlled Trials, J Gen Intern Med, 31, 1, 109-116

[23] Turner-McGrievy GM et al, 2015, Comparative effectiveness of plant-based diets for weight loss: A randomized controlled trial of five different diets, Nutrition, 31, 2, 350-358

[24] Dinu M et al, 2017, Vegetarian, vegan diets and multiple health outcomes: A systematic review with meta-analysis of observational studies, Crit Rev Food Sci Nutr, 57, 17, 3640-3549

[25] Satija A. 2018, Changes in intake of plant-based diets and weight change among men and women in the US, Presented at the American Society for Nutrition Scientific Sessions and Annual Meeting, June 9-12, 2018; Boston

[26] Piotr KK et al, 2017, Life with a Gastric Band. Long-Term Outcomes of Laparoscopic Adjustable Gastric Banding—a Retrospective Study, Obes Surg, 27, 5, 1250-1253

[27] https://asmbs.org/resources/studies-weigh-in-on-safety-and-effectiveness-of-newer-bariatric-and-metabolic-surgery-procedure

[28] Togerson JS et al, 2014, Xenical in the prevention of diabetes in obese subjects (XENDOS) study: a randomised study of orlistat as an adjunct to lifestyle changes for the prevention of type 2 diabetes in obese patients, Diabetes Care, 27, 1, 155-61

[29] Hollywood A and Ogden J, 2014, Gaining weight after taking orlistat: A qualitative study of patients at 18-months follow-up, J Health Psychol, 21, 5, 590-8

[30] Park KS, 2010, Raspberry ketone increases both lipolysis and fatty acid oxidation in 3Ts-L1 adipocytes, Planta Med, 76, 15, 1654-8.

[31] Hill S et al, 2014, The effect of non-caloric sweeteners on cognition, choice and post-consumption satisfaction, Appetite, 83, 82-88

[32] Swithers SE, Davidson RL, 2008, A role for sweet taste: calorie predictive relations in energy regulation in rats, Behav Neurosci, 122, 1, 161-73

[33] Hazuda H et al, presented at the American Diabetes Association's Scientific Sessions, San Diego, 2011.

[34] Swithers SE, 2013, Artificial sweeteners produce the counterintuitive effect of inducing metabolic derangements, Trends Endocrinol Metab, 24, 9, 431-41

[35] Shai I et al, 2008, Weight loss with a low-carbohydrate, Mediterranean, or low-fat diet. N Engl J Med, 359, 3, 229-41.

[36] Wardle J, Beales S, 1988, Control and loss of control over eating: An experimental investigation, J Abnorm Psychol, 97, 1, 35-40.

[37] Vatansever-Ozen S et al, 2011, The effects of exercise on food intake and hunger: relationship with acylated ghrelin and leptin, J Sports Sci Med, 10, 2, 283-291

[38] Patel SR et al, 2006, Association between reduced sleep and weight gain in women. Am J Epidemiol, 164, 10, 947-54

[39] Eyre H et al, 2004, Preventing cancer, cardiovascular disease and diabetes: A common agenda for the American Cancer Society, the American Diabetes Association and the American Heart Association, CA: A Cancer Journal for Clinicians, 54, 4, 190-207.

[40] Melkani GC, Panda S, 2017, Time-restricted feeding for prevention and treatment of cardiometabolic disorders. J Physiol, 595, 12, 3691-3700

[41] Gill S, Panda S, 2015, A Smartphone App Reveals Erratic Diurnal Eating Patterns in Humans that Can Be Modulated for Health Benefits, Cell Metab, 22, 5, 789-98

[42] Pezzuto JM, 2008, Grapes and human health: a perspective, J Agric Food Chem, 56, 16, 6777-84

[43] Zern TL et al, 2005, Grape polyphenols exert a cardioprotective effect in pre- and postmenopausal women by lowering plasma lipids and reducing oxidative stress J Nutr, 135, 8, 1911-7

[44] Singh CK et al, 2015, Resveratrol, in its natural combination in whole grape, for health promotion and disease management, Ann NY Acad Sci, 1348, 1, 150-160

[45] Ostman EM et al, 2001, Inconsistency between glycemic and insulinemic responses to regular and fermented milk products, Am J Clin Nutr, 74, 1, 96-100

[46] Liljeberg E et al, 2001, Milk as a supplement to mixed meals may elevate postprandial insulinemia, Eur J clin Nutr, 55, 11, 994-9.

[47] Siri-Tarino PW et al, 2010, Meta-analysis of prospective cohort studies evaluating the association of saturated fat with cardiovascular disease, Am J Clin Nutr, 91, 3, 535-46

[48] Hession M et al, 2009, Systematic review of randomized controlled trials of low-carbohydrate vs. low-fat/low-calorie diets in the management of obesity and its comorbidities. Obes Rev, 10, 1, 36-50.

[49] https://www.nhs.uk/live-well/eat-well/eat-less-saturated-fat/

[50] de Roos NM et al, 2003, Trans fatty acids, HDL-cholesterol, and cardiovascular disease. Effects of dietary changes on vascular reactivity, Eur J Med Res, 8, 8, 355-7.

[51] https://webcommunities.hse.gov.uk/connect.ti/pesticidesforum/view?objectId=49875

[52] Maruti S, et al, 2008, A prospective study of bowel motility and related factors on breast cancer risk, Cancer Epid Biomarkers Prev, 17 7, 1746-1750.

[53] Christensen TF, 2009, A Physiological Model of the Effect of Hypoglycemia on Plasma Potassium, J Diabetes Sci Technol, 3, 4, 887-894

[54] Drake SL, Drake MA, 2011, Comparison of salty taste and time intensity of sea and land salts from around the world, J Sensory Studies, 26, 1, 25-34

[55] Swithers SE, Davidson RL, 2008, A role for sweet taste: calorie predictive relations in energy regulation in rats, Behav Neurosci, 122, 1, 161-73

[56] Feijo Fde M et al, 2013, Saccharin and aspartame, compared with sucrose, induce greater weight gain in adult Wistar rats, at similar total caloric intake levels, Appetite, 60, 1, 203-7

[57] Azad MB et al, 2017, Nonnutritive sweeteners and cardiometabolic health: a systematic review and meta-analysis of randomized controlled trials and prospective cohort studies, CMAJ, 189, 28, E929-E939

[58] Suez J et al, 2014, Artificial sweeteners induce glucose intolerance by altering the gut microbiota. Nature, 514, 181-186

[59] Diamant M et al, 2011, Do nutrient-gut-microbiota interactions play a role in human obesity, insulin resistance and type 2 diabetes? Obes Rev, 12, 4, 272-81

[60] Cani PD, Delzenne NM, 2009, The role of the gut microbiota in energy metabolism and metabolic disease. Curr Pharm Des , 15, 13, 1546-58

[61] Stahl T et al, 2017, Migration of aluminium from food contact materials to food-a health risk for consumers? Part I of III: exposure to aluminium, release of aluminium, tolerable weekly intake (TWI), toxicological effects of aluminium, study design, and methods. Environ Sci Eur, 29, 1, 19

[62] Betts KS, 2007, Perfluoroalkyl acids: what is the evidence telling us? Environ Health Perspect, 115, 5, A250-256

[63] https://pubchem.ncbi.nlm.nih.gov/compound/Pentadecafluorooctanoic_acid#section= Top

[64] Aune D et al, 2017, Fruit and vegetable intake and the risk of cardiovascular disease, total cancer and all-cause mortality-a systematic review and dose-response meta-analysis of prospective studies, Int J Epidemiol, 46, 3, 1029-1056

[65] Li L, Seeram NP, 2011, Further investigation into maple syrup yields 3 new lignans, a new phenylpropanoid, and 26 other phytochemicals., J Agric Food Chem, 59, 14, 7708-16.

[66] https://www.nhs.uk/conditions/fluoride/

[67] https://www.nhs.uk/conditions/fluoride/

[68] https://www.nhs.uk/live-well/exercise/

[69] Sigal RJ et al, 2007, Effects of aerobic training, resistance training or both on glycemic control in type 2 diabetes: a randomised trial, Ann Intern Med, 147, 6, 357-69

[70] https://www.nhs.uk/live-well/exercise/

[71] Bernstein L, 1994, Physical exercise and reduced risk of breast cancer in young women, J Natl Cancer Inst, 86, 18, 1403-8.

[72] Lahmann PH et al, 2007, Physical activity and breast cancer risk: the European Prospective Investigation into Cancer and Nutrition, Cancer Epidemiol Biomarkers Prev, 16, 1, 36-42

[73] Johnston CS, 2005, Strategies for healthy weight loss: from vitamin C to the glycemic response, J Am Coll Nutr, 24, 3,158-165

[74] The Independent Food Commission's Food Magazine 2005

[75] Sakhaee K et al (1999), Meta-analysis of calcium bioavailability: a comparison of calcium citrate with calcium carbonate, Am J Ther, 5, 313-321.

[76] Linde K et al, 2008, St John's wort for major depression, Cochrane Database Syst Rev, 8, 4, CD000448

[77] Woelk H, 2000, Comparison of St John's wort and imipramine for treating depression: randomised controlled trial, British Medical Journal, 321, 7260, 536-539

[78] Cuomo A et al, 2017, Depression and Vitamin D Deficiency: Causality, Assessment, and Clinical Practice Implications, Neuropsychiatry, 7, 5,

[79] Jorde R et al, 2008, Effects of vitamin D supplementation on symptoms of depression in overweight and obese subjects: randomized double blind trial, J Intern Med, 264, 6, 599-609

[80] Darup D et al, 2012, A reverse J-shaped association of all-cause mortality with serum 25-hydroxyvitamin D in general practice: the CopD study, J Clin Endocrinol, Metab, 97, 8, 2644-52

[81] Hyponnen E et al, 2009, Serum 25-hydroxyvitamin D and IgE - a significant but nonlinear relationship. Allergy, 54, 4, 613-620

[82] Peet M et al, 1998, Depletion of omega-3 fatty acid levels in red blood cell membranes of depressive patients, Bio Psychiatry, 43, 5, 315-9

[83] Martins JG, 2009, EPA but not DHA appears to be responsible for the efficacy of omega-3 long chain polyunsaturated fatty acid supplementation in depression: evidence from a meta-analysis of randomized controlled trials, J Am Coll Nutr, 28, 5, 525-42

[84] Shaw K et al, 2002, Tryptophan and 5-hydroxytryptophan for depression, Cochrane Database Syst Rev. 2002;(1):CD003198.

[85] Ng TP et al, 2009, Folate, vitamin B12, homocysteine, and depressive symptoms in a population sample of older Chinese adults, J Am Geriatr Soc, 57, 5, 871-6

[86] Segal ZV et al, 2010, Antidepressant monotherapy vs sequential pharmacotherapy and mindfulness-based cognitive therapy, or placebo, for relapse prophylaxis in recurrent depression, Arch Gen Psychiatry, 67, 12, 1256-64

[87] Abenavoli L et al, 2010, Milk thistle in liver diseases: past, present, future, Phytother Res, 24, 10, 1423-32

[88] The Effect of Artichoke Leaf Extract on Alanine Aminotransferase and Aspartate Aminotransferase in the Patients with Nonalcoholic Steatohepatitis

[89] Panahi Y et al, 2018, Efficacy of artichoke leaf extract in non-alcoholic fatty liver disease: A pilot double-blind randomized controlled trial. Phytother Res, 32, 7, 1382-1387

[90] Hirsch A and Gomez R, 1995, Weight reduction through intalation of odoorants, J Neurol Orthop Med Sufl, 16, 28-31

[91] Schieberle P et al, 2009-2012, Identifying substances that regulate satiety in oils and fats and improving low-fat foodstuffs by adding lipid compounds with a high satiety effect; Key findings of the DFG/AiF cluster project "Perception of fat content and regulating satiety: an approach to developing low-fat foodstuffs", 2009-2012.

[92] Shen J et al, 2005, Olfactory stimulation with scent of grapefruit oil affects autonomic nerves, lipolysis and appetite in rats. Neurosci Lett, 380, 3, 289-94

[93] Ejaz A et al, 2009, Curcumin inhibits adipogenesis in 3T3-L1 adipocytes and angiogenesis and obesity in C57/BL mice, J Nutr, 139, 5, 919-925.

[94] Whiting S et al, 2014, Could capsaicinoids help to support weight management? A systematic review and meta-analysis of energy intake data, Appetite, 73, 183-188

[95] Hursel R, Westerterp-Plantenga MS, 2010, Thermogenic ingredients and body weight regulation, Int J Obes (Lond), 34, 4, 659-69

[96] Zare R et al, 2014, Effect of cumin powder on body composition and lipid profile in overweight and obese women, Complement Ther Clin Pract, 20, 4, 297-310

[97] Taghizadeh M et al, 2015, Effect of the cumin cyminum L. Intake on Weight Loss, Metabolic Profiles and Biomarkers of Oxidative Stress in Overweight Subjects: A Randomized Double-Blind Placebo-Controlled Clinical Trial, Ann Nutri Metab, 66 (2-3), 117-24

[98] Rahman MM et al, 2017, Cardamom powder supplementation prevents obesity, improves glucose intolerance, inflammation and oxidative stress in liver of high carbohydrate high fat diet induced obese rats, Lipids Health Dis, 16, 1, 151

[99] European Society of Human Genetics (ESHG). "Revolutionizing diets, improving health with discovery of new genes involved in food preferences." ScienceDaily, 1 June 2014.

Index

Printed in Great Britain
by Amazon

79930780R00102